# Nature's Aphrodisiacs

# Nature's Aphrodisiacs

by
**Nancy L. Nickell**

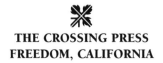

THE CROSSING PRESS
FREEDOM, CALIFORNIA

*Thanks to…*
*My husband, Joe, and daughter, Michelle,*
*for their encouragement and patience.*

*Vincent and Tatiana Capraro,*
*the harbingers of good fortune.*

*Jill Schettler and Beth Petro Roybal,*
*who brought this book to fruition.*

This book is designed to provide information in regard to the subject matter covered. It is sold with the understanding that the publisher and author are not engaged in rendering medical or other professional services. If medical or any other expert assistance is required, the services of a physician should be sought.

For information on bulk purchases or group discounts for this and other Crossing Press titles, please contact our Special Sales Manager at 800/777-1048.

Visit our Web site: www.crossingpress.com

**Library of Congress Cataloging-in-Publication Data**
Nickell, Nancy L.
  Nature's aphrodisiacs / Nancy L. Nickell.
    p. cm.
  Includes index.
  ISBN 0-89594-890-7
  1. Aphrodisiacs.  2. Naturopathy.  I. Title.
  RM386 .N53    1999
  615'.766--dc21                                                    98-47924
                                                                         CIP

# Contents

# CHAPTER ONE

# *Legendary Aphrodisiacs, Fact or Fiction?*

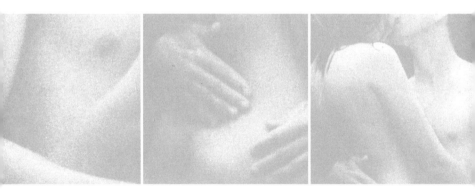

*T*hroughout the ages, men and women have eagerly swallowed almost any substance that was called an aphrodisiac, no matter how unappetizing or bizarre. In our never-ending search for better sex, humans have consumed such diverse items as oysters, onions, eels, elephant tusks, lion blood, ginseng, ginkgo, bull testicles, tiger blood, rhinoceros horn, ram penis, pig genitals, poison nuts, asparagus, alcohol, ambergris, mushrooms, marijuana, mandrake root, and the dried remains of the Mediterranean cantharis beetle, otherwise known as "Spanish fly."

The sea is a rich source of legendary aphrodisiacs. Oysters, shrimp, clams, anchovies, and eels have been reputed since ancient times to increase sexual desire. Indeed, the word "aphrodisiac" comes from Aphrodite, the Greek goddess of love and desire, who herself was a gift from the sea.

Many roots, vegetables, and fruits became known as aphrodisiacs simply because their shapes resemble human genitals. Surely those shapes were designed by nature as a clue to their use! So reasoned the ancients, who were always on the alert for such secret signs. Thus, based on shape alone, they chose to eat asparagus, bananas, beets, carrots, celery, cucumbers, dates, onions, garlic, mushrooms, tomatoes, turnips, and the vanilla bean, among others, in the hope that they would arouse passion or bestow sexual vigor. Ginseng is another example. Because the ginseng root is shaped like a man—with a torso, two legs, and two arms—people concluded that eating it would increase virility.

A group of plants that includes okra and fenugreek became known as aphrodisiacs because their juice is mucus-like. The ancients interpreted this as a sign that eating these plants would increase semen production.

Eating the genitals of animals noted for their potency, such as bulls and rams, is another historical practice meant to ensure virility.

# ❧ THE TRUTH BEHIND THE FICTION

Are these substances of folklore really aphrodisiacs? As it turns out, some of them do work as sex boosters, though their effects may not be as immediate or dramatic as hoped. Others work because the user believes they will work. Some, such as "Spanish fly," are dangerous. Others, while not harmful to people, are responsible for the slaughter of endangered animal species.

Ginseng is one of the legendary aphrodisiacs whose reputation has withstood the tests of time and of science. It has been used for fifty centuries or more as a tonic for energizing and rebuilding the whole body. Ginseng contains substances that work over time to increase libido, sexual responsiveness, and stamina. So do oysters, a prime source of zinc, one of the essential minerals for men. Semen is rich in zinc, and adequate zinc is needed for sperm production and hormone metabolism.

In the same way, shrimp turns out to be an important source of iodine, which is needed by the thyroid gland. The thyroid is the body's thermostat, the gland that regulates energy used to maintain body functions, including sex.

Through centuries of plant use and observation people learned that eating certain plants, seeds, and roots gave them added energy and sexual vigor. We now know that many of these plants are rich sources of vitamin E, the vitamin essential for reproduction. Similarly, certain vegetables considered to be aphrodisiacs are especially rich sources of vitamins and minerals. Mustard, garlic, onions, and leeks are rich in beneficial sulfur, for example.

In short, many substances used through the centuries as aphrodisiacs worked because they are natural tonics that stimulate good health and the optimum functioning of the reproductive system.

## ∾ STRICTLY SUPERSTITION

Some legendary aphrodisiacs should have remained the stuff of legends. If they seem to work, it is simply through the power of suggestion, and any effects are temporary. Some of these unproductive aphrodisiacs are:

- Cubeb (*Piper cubeba*)
- Ergot (*Claviceps purpurea*)
- Nux vomica (*Strychnos nux-vomica*)
- Sanguinaria, or bloodroot (*Sanguinaria canadensis*)
- Wild lettuce, or lettuce opium (*Latauca virosa*)

One herb, hops, has the unusual property of reducing sex drive in men but increasing it in women. Hops contains the female hormone estrogen and is a sexual stimulant for women but a sedative for men.

## ∾ FROM SUPERSTITION TO SCIENCE

Which of nature's legendary aphrodisiacs really work? Unfortunately, little clinical research has been done on the subject. In fact, only two herbal substances—*yohimbine* and *muira puama*—have been clinically tested and proven to be effective aphrodisiacs. A third herb, *damiana*, contains an essential oil that stimulates the genital tract and alkaloids that can increase sensitivity of the sexual organs. Although it has been chemically analyzed in the laboratory and shown to contain substances that increase sexual arousal, damiana has not been tested in clinical trials.

Why has so little research been done in a field that is admittedly so fascinating? The answer is a familiar one—money. Today most drug research is conducted by major pharmaceutical companies, which depend on patents for profits.

You can't patent a carrot or an herb. This explains why the research on yohimbine and muira puama, for example, was conducted by non-profit organizations. Most of the evidence we have on aphrodisiacs that work is anecdotal. The powers of these aphrodisiacs have been attested to by generations of users through the centuries. Although such evidence is not scientific, it is substantial, and should not be ignored.

## CHAPTER TWO

*Aphrodisiacs and
The Stages of Sexual Response*

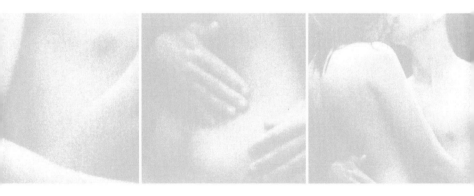

*I*n 1966, pioneering researchers William H. Masters and Virginia E. Johnson published *Human Sexual Response*, a groundbreaking, thoroughly researched book on how men and women respond to sexual stimulation. Masters and Johnson described sexual response as a four-stage cycle: *excitement*, *plateau*, *orgasm*, and *resolution*.

Later, a modified version was worked out by another sex researcher and therapist, Helen Singer Kaplan. Her model includes the psychological and emotional components of sexual arousal and consists of three stages: *desire*, *arousal*, and *orgasm*. As a sex therapist, Kaplan worked with a number of patients who had problems with sexual arousal. This led her to conclude that some people do not have much desire to be sexually aroused. Thus she introduced *desire* as the first stage in sexual response. The second stage, *arousal*, is characterized by a buildup of blood (vasocongestion) in the pelvic area and an increasing muscular tension throughout the body. This causes the heart rate, breathing rate, and blood pressure to increase. The third stage, *orgasm*, releases muscle tension and vasocongestion, and gradually all bodily functions return to their normal level.

Aphrodisiacs can help all three levels of the sexual response. There are aphrodisiacs that increase *desire*. Many herbs and aromatic oils, for example, increase desire by creating moods and emotions conducive to lovemaking. Certain amino acids increase desire by boosting neurotransmitter levels in the brain. This facilitates reactions to sensual stimuli, contributing to the brain's creation of sexual thoughts and fantasies, and its transmission of chemical messages that activate sexual arousal.

Aphrodisiacs of all types contribute to the *arousal* stage—herbs, foods and nutrients, pheromones, aromatic oils, and neurotransmitter and hormone boosters. Some, for example, promote vasocongestion in the genitals and facilitate erections. Others affect hormones that trigger lubrication of the vagina and skin sensitivity. Still others work to maintain long-term sexual energy and vigor.

The third stage, *orgasm*, depends on the efficient functioning of many body systems as well as the psychological and emotional capacity to temporarily put aside problems and distractions and enjoy having sex. Nature's aphrodisiacs can come to the rescue, boosting both the physiological and psychological aspects of sex.

In brief, nature *does* produce aphrodisiacs—natural substances that enhance sexual desire, arousal, and performance—though these are not necessarily the same substances that have been considered aphrodisiacs through the ages. Today's surge of interest in complementary medicine, including such areas as aromatherapy and *phyto* (plant) chemicals, has contributed substantially to our knowledge of nature's aphrodisiacs. Science has made its contributions, too, especially in research on how pheromones, neurotransmitters, and hormones affect sexual activity.

When people speak of aphrodisiacs they usually mean substances that work immediately to arouse sexual desire. Usually these substances affect the genitals directly—either by increasing blood flow to those areas or increasing their sensitivity. Such aphrodisiacs are usually taken just prior to lovemaking. But there are a myriad of substances that enhance sex in other ways and that have a longer-lasting effect, reinforcing sexual arousal and response. Some boost the physical aspects of sex; others create moods and emotions conducive to sexual activity and romance.

The forces that regulate sexual arousal are both mental and physical. Sexual arousal may be triggered mentally—by thoughts and fantasies, reading an erotic book, talking about sex, or reacting to a provocative sexual remark. It may be triggered by purely visual stimuli—a sexually attractive person, an erotic movie, nonverbal body messages, or nudity. Or it may be stimulated by messages from the other senses—hearing a sexy voice, smelling an evocative fragrance, or being touched. Sexual arousal is usually triggered consciously, but it can occur involuntarily. The phenomena of nocturnal emissions and of orgasms for both men and women during sleep appear to be examples of involuntary sexual arousal. These events usually occur during the REM (rapid eye movement) stage of sleep, when dreaming also occurs. It seems logical to suspect that they result from erotic dreams, but when men in clinical studies were awakened when they had an erection and asked about what they were dreaming, they seldom reported an erotic dream.

Both men's and women's genitals go through automatic, measurable episodes of arousal during REM sleep—approximately once every ninety minutes. The genitals are aroused along with other kinds of nervous system arousal (e.g., increased pulse, increased breathing rate, changes in eye movement, and changes in the skin's electrical resistance). According to June M. Reinisch and Ruth Beasley in *The Kinsey Institute New Report on Sex*, no one is sure why these sexual responses occur. One theory is that the body is running a test of its systems to see if everything is in working order. The human sexual response is complex, involving a number of bodily systems. It is ultimately controlled by the brain, but also depends upon the proper functioning of the circulatory system, muscles, nervous system, neurotransmitters, endocrine glands, and hormones.

How is all of this related to aphrodisiacs? Sexual arousal and response can be triggered in many ways—both mental and physical—and require the proper functioning of the body's systems. The body's biochemistry plays a huge role in the functioning of those systems as well as in the functioning of the brain itself—the ultimate controller of the sex drive. And our biochemistry is tremendously influenced by the substances we consume. Whether they are foods, drugs, herbs, vitamins, minerals, amino acids, phyto (plant) hormones, or aromatic oils, all of these "chemical" substances affect our biochemistry, and hence our sexuality. In this book I discuss aphrodisiacs that work on all of these bodily systems.

# CHAPTER THREE

## *Herbs as Aphrodisiacs*

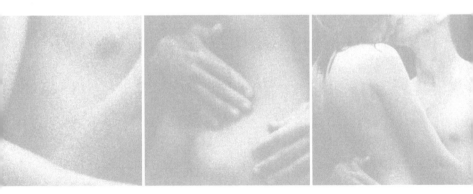

*T*here are many herbs that act as aphrodisiacs although they work in a variety of ways for different results. Fast-acting herbs are taken prior to having sex and can affect one or a combination of the stages of sexual response. These aphrodisiacs can have physical effects (such as increasing blood flow to the genitals), emotional effects (such as relieving stress and anxiety), or both.

There are other herbal aphrodisiacs that work long-term on our overall constitution and specific body systems. Taken regularly over a period of time, these herbs provide us with physical and emotional readiness for long-term sexual desire, energy, vigor, and function.

Whatever herbs you take, it is important to understand how to take them for maximum effectiveness and safety. Unlike pharmaceuticals, herbs and herbal preparations vary in strength and effectiveness depending on such variables as where the herbs were grown, when they were harvested, and how they were processed and stored. Thus suggested dosages are not standardized as they are for pharmaceuticals. In this chapter suggested doses are given where that information is available, but these should only be used as general guidelines. It is safest to start with a low dosage. Then if needed, slowly increase your intake.

Labels on herbal preparations provide information on dosages. An herbalist, if available, can help you determine your individual requirements. When taking herbs it is best to start slowly and to pay attention to what your body is telling you. This will help you avoid adverse reactions. Keep in mind, however, that many herbs take time to effect a change. Be patient. Don't rush headlong into increasing your dosage on the theory that "more is better." With herbs, balance is the key.

## ❧ HERBS TAKEN PRIOR TO LOVEMAKING FOR PHYSICAL EFFECTS

Most fast-acting herbs increase physical arousal and sexual function of both men and women. For example, ginkgo, cayenne, and ginger help open the blood vessels that lead to the genitals. This increased blood flow facilitates erection and sexual performance in men and increases sexual sensations in both men and women. Three of these fast-acting herbs—damiana, muira puama, and yohimbine—are the only herbal aphrodisiacs that have been studied by researchers.

### Cayenne Pepper *(Capsicum frutescens)*
Cayenne pepper, also called red pepper, is well known as both an herb and a spice. When taken orally it increases circulation. It is also applied externally to stop bleeding and treat pain and inflammation. Cayenne pepper is made from the dried, ground fruit of various hot chili peppers. Its active ingredient is capsaicin, a substance that stimulates circulation and digestion.

Cayenne is sold in capsules, concentrated drops, and tinctures. As an aphrodisiac it is taken about thirty minutes prior to lovemaking. A dose is 10 to 15 drops of tincture or concentrated drops, or a 400–500 milligram (mg) capsule. It may also be prepared as a tea by pouring one cup of boiling water over one teaspoon of powdered cayenne. The dosage is one fluid ounce (1/8 cup) of tea.

### Damiana *(Turnera aphrodisiaca)*
Damiana is a small shrub native to North America. It can be found growing in dry, sandy, or rocky places in the American Southwest as far north as Texas. Damiana is used as an aphrodisiac by both sexes. In Mexico it was first used primarily by women, who drank damiana tea prior to lovemaking. Today it is used by women to treat low libido, urinary and vaginal

infections, and menstrual problems. Men use it as a remedy for impotence, premature ejaculation, and prostate complaints. Damiana is often combined with saw palmetto in formulas that treat impotency or problems of the prostate.

Although no clinical studies have been conducted on the effects of damiana, chemical analysis shows that damiana contains alkaloids similar to caffeine that have stimulating and aphrodisiacal effects. These alkaloids stimulate blood flow to the genital area and increase sensitivity. In addition to alkaloids, damiana contains a mildly irritating oil that stimulates the genitourinary tract. Damiana also helps regulate hormonal activity and calms the nerves. Some people experience a mild euphoria for several hours after taking damiana.

Damiana is available in capsule form, concentrated drops, and extracts. It is also an ingredient in many combination herbal formulas.

Other uses of damiana: To relieve depression, anxiety, exhaustion, constipation, digestive complaints, incontinence, water retention, and mucus congestion.

### Ginger *(Zingiber officinale)*

Ginger is derived from the root of the plant and is highly stimulating. It increases blood flow to the genitals of both men and women, stirring sexual sensations. Fresh ginger roots are sold in supermarkets and many health food stores. The roots may be grated and made into a tea, using 1 pint of boiling water to 1 1/2 tablespoons of grated ginger, and simmering for 7 minutes. Grated ginger may be placed in a plastic bag and frozen. It thaws quickly. Pickled ginger, available in the Asian food section of many grocery stores, is used as a condiment.

Ginger is also available dried and in tablets, capsules, concentrated drops, tinctures, and extracts. A dose is usually 500–1,000 mg of dried ginger or 1–2 droppersful of tincture or concentrated drops.

Ginger is a blood thinner and should not be used if you are taking prescription anticoagulant drugs or aspirin.

### Ginkgo *(Ginkgo biloba)*

Ginkgo promotes blood flow to the genitals by expanding the walls of the blood vessels. For best results it should be taken daily. (Its use as a long-term aphrodisiac is described in the next section.) When taken for a fast-acting aphrodisiac prior to lovemaking, the usual dosage is increased and taken an hour before sexual activity begins. For this use the recommended dosage is three 60 mg capsules or 30 drops of the liquid form taken sublingually (under the tongue).

Ginkgo is a blood thinner and should not be used if you are taking prescription anticoagulant drugs or aspirin.

### Kava Kava *(Piper methysticum)*

Kava kava can induce hallucinations and heighten sexuality. It evokes warmth and can stimulate the genitals. When used as an aphrodisiac, kava kava tea is drunk before having sex—but not more than an hour before. Otherwise the desire for sex will succumb to the desire for sleep. (See also pp. 28–29 for information on the emotional effects of kava kava.)

### Muira Puama *(Ptychopetalum olacoides)*

Muira puama, or "potency wood," has long been used by Brazilian and Peruvian Indians as a powerful aphrodisiac and nerve stimulant. Its use as an aphrodisiac has been documented in books since 1930. This long-term, documented use prompted Dr. Jacques Waynberg, a foremost authority on sexual function, to investigate muira puama. In 1995 he conducted a clinical study of the effectiveness of muira puama at the Institute of Sexology in Paris, France. He worked with 262 men who complained of lack of sexual desire and inability to attain or maintain an erection. The patients were given a daily dose of 1.4 grams of muira puama extract. Within two weeks, 62 percent of the patients with a low sexual drive claimed that muira puama had a dynamic effect; 51 percent of patients with erection problems said it was beneficial.

An article published in 1994 in *The American Journal of Natural Medicine* stated: "Preliminary research indicates one of the best herbs to use for erectile dysfunction or lack of libido may be muira puama (also known as potency wood)."

Muira puama tea is drunk a short time before lovemaking. The tea is made by boiling or steeping the root, or it may be made from a tincture of muira puama mixed with water. Like damiana, muira puama is often combined with other herbs in combination formulas.

Other uses of muira puama: For menstrual cramps and premenstrual syndrome; as a stimulant, stomach tonic, and treatment for rheumatism.

### Yohimbine

Yohimbine is derived from the bark of the yohimbe tree, an evergreen native to West Africa. Yohimbe bark has been eaten, sniffed, smoked, rubbed on the body, and made into a tea, all because of its powerful aphrodisiacal properties. Researchers discovered that the active ingredient in yohimbe is *yohimbine hydrochloride*, a crystalline alkaloid. Although it is possible to buy yohimbe bark, it is safer to use yohimbine hydrochloride. The amount of yohimbine contained in the yohimbe bark could vary, making it impossible to prescribe an accurate dose. For this reason, the FDA considers yohimbe (but not yohimbine hydrochloride) unsafe. It is yohimbine hydrochloride that is used in clinical studies and in drugs. In fact, yohimbine hydrochloride is the only FDA-approved herbal substance for treating certain types of male impotence. Yohimbine works by inducing dilation of certain blood vessels in the penis. It also increases release of norepinephrine, a neurotransmitter that is helpful in producing erections.

Yohimbine first began to be recognized by the public in the 1980s as a result of a strictly controlled study by researchers at Queen's University Medical School in Canada. Their study showed that yohimbine could help restore potency for diabetics and heart patients (who often have impotency problems). Their success rate was 44 percent, an impressive percentage for such patients. The results were reported in *Science Digest*, *Time*, and *Health*.

Additional studies have borne out the conclusions reached by the Canadian researchers. Several pharmaceutical companies have formulated prescription drugs that contain yohimbine. Examples include Yocon, Actibine, Aphrodyne, and Yohimex.

Yohimbine is stronger than either muira puama and damiana, but its side effects often make it impractical to use. According to Dr. Julian Davidson, who conducted a study on yohimbine at Stanford University, "Yohimbine does help men get an erection, but they don't know what to do with it because they feel so lousy."

Yohimbine should be used only under the guidance of a physician. It should not be used by individuals with kidney disease, high blood pressure, or psychological problems.

Side effects may include: elevated blood pressure and heart rate, nausea, stomach pain, diarrhea, dizziness, headaches, skin flushing, hallucinations, anxiety attacks, and panic attacks.

Yohimbine must *never* be taken with food or substances that contain *tyramine*, an amino acid. To do so may cause hypertension (high blood pressure). For example, do not take yohimbine with liver, cheese, red wine, and certain diet aids and decongestants.

## ❧ HERBS TAKEN PRIOR TO LOVEMAKING FOR EMOTIONAL EFFECTS

Sex is more than hormones, and sexual desire is ignited—or squelched—by signals other than the purely physical. The mind and emotions exert a powerful influence over sex, both to arouse sexual desire and to extinguish it. Lack of confidence, stress, worry, anxiety, depression, fear of failure, anger—all these and more can deflate sex drive and impair performance. Negative emotions such as depression or performance anxiety (excessive worry about sexual performance) create body chemicals that can cause impotency.

No matter how healthy your hormones, how active your glands, when you are emotionally down your sex life will suffer. Psychological blocks to sex are real. Fortunately, they need not be permanent. One way to attack them is through herbs that ease tension and elevate mood.

### *Angelica* (*Angelica archangelica*)
Angelica received its name from a legend that arose during the time of the bubonic plague. According to the legend, an angel appeared in a dream and revealed that the herb was a treatment for the plague. Thus the herb came to be called "angelica," or "the root of the Holy Ghost." Besides being an aphrodisiac, angelica also has the ability to relieve headaches caused by nervous tension. If bedtime headaches are a recurring problem, try drinking angelica tea at night as a preventive measure.

Other uses of angelica: To regulate the menstrual cycle, improve circulation, relieve spasms of the bowels and stomach, and relieve heartburn.

Angelica is a strong emmenagogue (brings on the menses, or period). It should not be used by pregnant women.

Diabetics should avoid using angelica. It contains sugars.

### Gotu Kola *(Centella asiatica)*

Gotu kola is considered to be an excellent nerve tonic. It stimulates the central nervous system, decreases depression and fatigue, and stimulates the sex drive. Taken regularly, gotu kola tea reportedly has a cumulative effect as a sex-drive booster. The Chinese say that two leaves of gotu kola a day keep old age away.

Gotu kola is a good long-term approach to combating nervousness and tension. It is a safe, long-term, herbal "upper." Unlike caffeine-containing herbs, gotu kola does not cause insomnia, nervousness, restlessness, or anxiety. Rather, it promotes a sense of well-being, and in large doses has a calming effect. Gotu kola promotes mental calm and clarity, improves memory, and alleviates insomnia.

Other uses of gotu kola: To treat mental and neurological disturbances, high blood pressure, urinary tract infections, and hepatitis.

Excessive doses of gotu kola can cause headaches or fainting.

### Kava Kava *(Piper methysticum)*

Kava kava (also called kava) is a mildly narcotic but legal drink from the South Pacific, where it has been used in traditional ceremonies for at least three thousand years. In one ceremony, men form a large circle. A female virgin stands in the center of the circle, chews a kava root, and then spits it into a coconut shell. This is mixed with water and the men drink it. The result is euphoria and, they claim, the ability to attain a higher level of consciousness and communicate with the gods.

The active ingredients in kava kava are narcotic substances called alpha pyrones. These pyrones can relax muscles and depress the nervous system. The result is a state of relaxed euphoria. Kava kava reduces anxiety and nervousness and promotes a pleasant, warm, and sociable feeling of well-being.

In the islands of the South Pacific fresh kava kava root is fermented to make an alcoholic beverage that is drunk during social rituals and to relax tension between disputing parties. A few cups induce a short-term "high" accompanied by feelings of tranquillity and friendliness. Unlike alcoholic social drinking, kava kava does not affect the ability to think clearly. Although relaxed and happy, the kava kava drinker retains mental clarity and alertness. If the drinker falls into a kava-induced sleep, it is a deep, dreamless sleep that is followed by mental clarity, not a hangover. Today kava kava is called the official drink of the Pacific, and there are kava bars in Fiji and Polynesia.

The kava kava roots most valued as aphrodisiacs are those that are at least twenty years old. The huge, gnarled roots attain this age near sea level in places like Samoa, Tahiti, and Fiji. These roots can weigh up to a hundred pounds. Since the root is not soluble in water, it is either beaten and mashed into minute pieces that are mixed with water or fermented to make an alcoholic beverage.

In North America kava kava root is usually available only in its dried form, which must be mashed in a blender or food processor. Occasionally it is sold as an extract that can be mixed with water to make tea.

Other uses of kava kava: To relieve pain, treat headaches and migraines, lose weight, relieve fatigue, combat insomnia, and eliminate water retention.

Kava kava is a mild narcotic and is habit forming.

Very large doses may result in impaired driving ability.

It should not be used by those with Parkinson's disease or by those taking benzodiazepines (antidepressants).

### *Lemon Balm* (*Melissa officinalis*)

Lemon balm (or bee balm) is a type of mint plant native to Europe. Lemon balm is very soothing. It relaxes the nervous system and is mildly sedative, but it also elevates mood. In *The Historie of Plants*, written in 1597, John Gerard states, "It maketh the heart merry and joyful and strengtheneth the vitall spirits."

Drinking lemon balm tea to alleviate stress and frayed nerves is customary in Europe. It is one of the most gentle and pleasant-tasting of the calming herbs.

Other uses of lemon balm: To relieve stomach distress, combat insomnia, lower high blood pressure, and regulate the menstrual cycle.

Avoid using lemon balm if you have a thyroid condition. Lemon balm may interfere with a hormone that stimulates the thyroid.

### Skullcap *(Scutellaria lateriflora)*
Skullcap is a tranquilizing herb, very useful for relieving any stress or nervousness associated with having sex. It is a safe, mild herb that relaxes the nervous system and muscular tension and induces inner calm. Skullcap is native to North America, where it can be found in swampy woods and marshes. Traditionally, skullcap has been used to treat anxiety, insomnia, and withdrawal from barbiturates and tranquilizers.

Other uses of skullcap: To relieve menstrual cramps and muscle spasms, to promote suppressed menstruation.

Skullcap should not be taken by pregnant women.

When used in excess, skullcap can cause dizziness, stupor, and confusion.

### Valerian *(Valeriniana officinalis)*
Valerian is native to Europe but is now found across the northern United States and into Canada. Its dry, powdered root is the most widely used calming herb in Europe. In Germany, for example, there are more than a hundred over-the-counter preparations that contain valerian.

Valerian root has components called "valepotriates" that chemically relax tense nerves and help alleviate anxiety. Valerian has marvelous stress-reducing properties. It is also a mild sedative. In 1989 Drs. Holzl and Goau of the Institute of Pharmaceutical Biology in Marburg, Germany, discovered that valerian acts as a sedative in a similar, but much milder, way to a group of drugs called benzodiazepines, of which Valium is the best-known example. Unlike synthetic drugs, however, valerian does not cause addiction or dependence. When used to treat insomnia, valerian does not cause a hangover or impaired concentration the next day as do prescription drugs like Halcion.

Because of its safety and its effectiveness in treating stress and anxiety, healthcare professionals consider valerian the natural treatment of choice for anxiety or insomnia.

Valerian has only one drawback. It smells like sweaty socks or sneakers. Its taste is similar to its smell. For this reason, valerian is often taken in capsule form.

Other uses of valerian: To treat ulcers, headaches, colic, intestinal gas, muscle cramps, and muscle spasms.

Although valerian is not addictive, it should not be taken in large doses or on a daily basis for long periods of time. Extended usage causes some people to be stimulated rather than calmed. While taking sedative drugs or antidepressants only take valerian under the supervision of a healthcare professional.

### Vervain (Verbena officinalis)
Vervain was one of seven sacred herbs of the druids, the Celtic priests and priestesses of pre-Christian Gaul and the British Isles. It was also sacred to the Romans, who tied it in bundles and used it to sweep and purify their altars. According to Ellen Evert Hopman in *A Druid's Herbal*, "Wearing or bathing in vervain places one under the influence of Diana. After washing your hands in the infusion, it will be possible to engender love in the one you touch."

A more reliable use of vervain for aphrodisiacal purposes is based on its ability to dispel nervousness and promote relaxation. Vervain tea is an herbal remedy for depression, nervous exhaustion, strain, stress, tension, and headaches. Chinese researchers have found that vervain is linked to dilation of arteries in the brain. This helps explain why vervain can relieve headaches, including migraines.

Vervain not only elevates the spirits, but also aids the detoxifying action of the liver. The ancient Celts believed that it purges calculi, or stones, from the bladder. The word "vervain" is Celtic, and is derived from *fer* (to drive away) and *faen* (stone).

Other uses of vervain: To increase breast milk, regulate the menstrual cycle, and treat eczema, colds, flu, coughs, and upper respiratory inflammation.

# ❧ HERBS TAKEN REGULARLY FOR LONG-TERM SEXUAL VIGOR

The herbs listed in this section enhance sex by gradually fortifying or stimulating the body's reproductive or hormonal systems or by combating depression. Many of them are said to increase energy levels and life span as well. Like most other easily obtainable natural substances, these long-term aphrodisiacs have not interested researchers from the pharmaceutical industry. Evidence that they work is primarily anecdotal, from long-time users.

## *Astragalus* *(Astragalus membranaceus)*

Astragalus (*huang chi*) is one of the most valued Chinese herbs. The American variety is sometimes called milk vetch. Astragalus boosts sex by energizing the body. It is a stimulant that steps up metabolism and adrenal gland function. Astragalus is especially useful as an energy builder for those aged thirty-five or younger who find that "once is enough."

Astragalus energizes the internal organs, helps regulate the nervous and hormonal systems, and boosts overall vitality. In addition, it stimulates the immune system. Herbalists recommend astragalus for those who have herpes. Taking astragalus during periods of stress helps to prevent recurring herpes attacks. Astragalus is available as an extract, a tea, and in capsules.

Other uses of astragalus: To build muscle tone, improve digestion, prevent cancer, reduce the adverse effects of chemotherapy, and lower the amount of chemotherapy drugs needed.

## *Black Cohosh* *(Cimicifuga racemosa)*

Black cohosh is an herb with a wide variety of uses, from strengthening the male sexual organ to repelling fleas. It is a perennial plant about 5 feet tall that is native to eastern North

America. Black cohosh is also known as black snakeroot, bug-bane, and rattleroot. According to folklore, its black cylindrical root can be used as an antidote for rattlesnake poison. The root of the plant is the part used for medicinal purposes. It is dried, cut up, and steeped or boiled to make a tea. Or it is used to make an extract or tincture. The flowers have an unusual, unpleasant odor that repels insects.

Black cohosh is used to strengthen both the male and female reproductive systems. It has a strong effect on the central nervous system and is used in many formulas designed to treat erection problems. An extract of the root was shown to strengthen the male reproductive organ in rats. Black cohosh contains a natural estrogen. Women use the herb to treat menstrual irregularities and the pains of childbirth.

Other uses of black cohosh: To treat rheumatism, high blood pressure, diarrhea, whooping cough, neuralgia, nervous conditions, fits, and convulsions.

### Burdock (Arctium lappa)

Burdock is a common, broad-leafed weed, three to four feet tall, with large dark leaves, purple flowers, and burrs. It is also known as beggar's burr, hardock, and thorny burr. In his *Complete Herbal*, published in 1694, Pechey wrote that burdock will "stir up lust." The Chinese use the root internally as an aphrodisiac and as an alternative treatment for syphilis.

Burdock is also used externally. Its powdered seeds and leaves are made into a salve to treat skin disorders. Its juice is rubbed into the scalp to fight baldness.

Other uses of burdock: Internally to treat arthritis, pro-statitis, urinary problems, sciatica, and lumbago. Externally to treat scrotal eczema, psoriasis, sebaceous cysts, boils, sties, carbuncles, and canker sores.

Burdock root is very potent. An overdose is toxic and will cause nausea and vomiting. It should be used with caution. It should be avoided by pregnant women.

## Chaste Tree *(Agnus castus)*
See Vitex.

## Coriander *(Coriandrum sativum)*
Coriander is usually thought of as an aromatic seasoning for soups and salads, but it has a more romantic side. Scheherazade, the narrator of *The Arabian Nights*, described coriander as an aphrodisiac in her tales. The druids made a lust potion by adding powdered coriander seeds to warm wine.

Coriander seeds are both stimulating and narcotic, which helps explain coriander's use as an aphrodisiac. The raw seeds are chewed to combat bad breath, but if used in large amounts the effect is narcotic.

Coriander is native to Europe, where its seeds are used for medicinal purposes. Fresh seeds have a noxious smell, but as they dry they become more and more fragrant. Their essential oil is used in aromatherapy.

Other uses of coriander: To treat indigestion, intestinal gas, diarrhea, and colic.

Coriander can be narcotic if used in great quantities.

## Cotton Root Bark *(Gossypium herbaceum)*
The cotton plant is native to India, but is still widely grown in the southern United States. The bark and root of the cotton plant are used to make a tea which, according to herbal folklore, is an aphrodisiac, and is said to have the power to cause abortion.

## Dong Quai *(Angelica sinensis)*
*Dong quai* is used by women to nourish the reproductive system and treat a variety of female complaints. Dong quai is a substance made from the root of the Chinese angelica plant (similar to the American variety of angelica). In China it has been used for generations to treat painful menstrual cramps and an irregular menstrual cycle. Today herbalists also use it

to treat symptoms of PMS (premenstrual syndrome), hot flashes and other symptoms of menopause, and symptoms caused by "going off the pill." Like ginseng, dong quai is considered to be a general tonic and strengthener that harmonizes vital energy.

Dong quai is rich in magnesium, vitamin $B_{12}$, and vitamin E, which nourish the nervous and reproductive systems. It also stimulates secretion of the female sex hormone estrogen. It is sold in health food stores as tablets, capsules, concentrated drops, tinctures, and extracts.

Other uses of dong quai: To lower blood pressure, reduce pain, improve circulation, and treat insomnia.

Pregnant women should avoid using dong quai.

### False Unicorn (Chamaelirium luteum)

False unicorn, or blazing star, is an excellent tonic for the genitourinary tract and is used for a variety of both female and male problems. Men take it to treat impotence and for problems with the urinary tract. Women use it to treat menstrual irregularity, nausea during pregnancy, and threatened miscarriage. It is also used to treat female hormone imbalance and infertility.

False unicorn is native to eastern North America. It is a perennial plant, about 19 inches high and grows in low, moist ground, meadows, thickets, and forests. The root of the plant is boiled to make tea.

Other uses of false unicorn: To eliminate intestinal parasites, to relieve stomach distress, as a diuretic, and as a stimulant.

If taken in large quantities, false unicorn causes vomiting. Overdosing is also dangerous for those with heart conditions. In large doses it can be a cardiac (heart) toxin.

### Fenugreek (Trigonella foenumgraecum)

Fenugreek has a long history as an aphrodisiac. Its use as a sexual stimulant began in ancient Egypt. The ancient Greek, Roman, and Ayurvedic (Indian) healers also used it as an aphrodisiac and to treat inflamed mucous membranes of the respiratory and digestive tract. In Turkey its powdered form is mixed with honey and eaten. Turkish men claim it increases sexual potency, and Turkish women say it strengthens their sex drive and sexual appeal.

Most likely it is the aromatic properties of fenugreek that heighten the user's sex appeal. Eating fenugreek sweetens the breath, decreases perspiration, and gives the body a sweet, maple-like aroma.

Fenugreek is native to Greece and other Mediterranean countries. Its seeds contain mucilage, which soothes the mucous membranes. They also contain estrogen-like substances that can benefit the female reproductive system. Fenugreek was an ingredient in the famous Victorian female remedy, Lydia Pinkham's Vegetable Compound. It is still used for menstrual pain and as a uterine tonic.

Other uses of fenugreek: To treat sore throats, bronchitis, colds, nasal congestion, allergies, asthma, emphysema, hay fever, heartburn, and migraine headaches.

Fenugreek may stimulate contractions of the uterus and should not be taken by pregnant women.

### Fo Ti *(Polygonum multiflorum)*

Fo ti is one of the most important herbs in Chinese medicine. In China, fo ti is used as a stimulant and tonic. It is said to strengthen sexual desire and performance, restore vitality, prevent premature aging, and rejuvenate the endocrine glands.

According to legend, fo ti's Chinese name, *he shou wu*, was the name of a Chinese man who regained sexual powers and longevity as a result of taking the herb. Childless and impotent, he began taking the herb at age fifty-eight. He became potent, fathered many children, and lived to the age of 130.

Fo ti is usually taken as a decoction, prepared by first soaking and then simmering the herb in water, and straining and drinking the liquid. In health food stores, fo ti is sold as a powder, tablets, capsules, concentrated drops, tincture, and extracts.

Other uses of fo ti: As a digestive tonic, as a diuretic, and to reduce cholesterol levels.

### Ginkgo *(Ginkgo biloba)*

The Chinese have been using the leaves and nuts of the ginkgo tree for thousands of years to increase sexual vitality, promote longevity, and treat a variety of ailments such as asthma, allergies, congested lungs, impaired hearing, cancer, and venereal disease. Until recently, ginkgo was largely ignored by the rest of the world, but now ginkgo is enjoying a worldwide surge of popularity because researchers have confirmed what the Chinese learned through generations of practical experience. Ginkgo contains chemical compounds that, over a period of time, produce remarkable effects on the human body.

One of these effects is its ability to improve the flow of blood to all vital tissues and organs of the body without increasing blood pressure. This amounts to an age-reversing process, because many conditions associated with aging are caused by impaired blood circulation. Decreased blood flow to the brain, for example, can cause impaired memory, forgetfulness, poor concentration, mental confusion, depression, and stroke. For this reason, ginkgo is being promoted as a "smart herb" and as a treatment for patients who suffer memory loss because of blocked blood vessels in the brain.

Because it increases blood flow to the genitals, ginkgo is also promoted as a sex-booster and as a treatment for impotence.

Ginkgo's effect is gradual; it may take months before results become noticeable. The recommended dose is a 60 mg capsule, or 10 drops of the liquid form taken sublingually, twice a day for at least a month. However, it is also taken prior to lovemaking to promote blood flow to the sexual organs. For this purpose, the dose is increased.

A clinical study reported in the *Journal of Urology* in 1989 concluded that ginkgo extract can help relieve impotence caused by insufficient blood supply to the penis. Sixty patients took part in the study. Each took a small dose of ginkgo (60 mg) daily for twelve to twenty-eight months. After six months, half of the patients had regained potency. Sonograms showed that blood flow to the penis increased after six to eight weeks.

In addition to improving blood circulation, ginkgo is an antioxidant. It protects cell membranes in the brain and other organs from damage by chemicals called "free radicals" that can destroy entire cells.

Ginkgo's reputation as an anti-aging herb is fitting, as ginkgo itself is probably the oldest variety of tree in existence. Charles Darwin called it "a living fossil." It is the only survivor of a plant species called ginkgoales, which lived over 200 million years ago in the age of the dinosaurs. Some ginkgo trees are over one thousand years old. The ginkgo tree is extremely hardy. A single ginkgo was the only tree to survive the atomic bomb blast in Hiroshima, Japan. It is resistant to insects, bacteria, viruses, and pollution.

Other uses of ginkgo: To treat hearing loss, ringing in the ears (tinnitus), impaired vision caused by retina damage, depression, cold hands and feet, migraine headaches, varicose veins, hemorrhoids, Alzheimer's disease, and dizziness.

### Ginseng *(Panax ginseng, Panax quinquefolius)*
Ginseng, the "king of herbs," is best known as an energizer, a revitalizer and—perhaps because of these properties—an aphrodisiac. Its name is Chinese and means literally "root, or essence, of man." Its therapeutic use in China dates back five thousand years. In the *Shennong Herbal*, compiled between the first and second centuries B.C., ginseng was listed as a superior medicine that could be used long-term without adverse effects. In the sixteenth century, the esteemed Asian physician Li Shih-chen recommended the ginseng root as an aphrodisiac and love potion, and to restore stamina for lovemaking.

Ginseng's use also dates back centuries in India, where it was prized for its ability to treat impotence. According to the ancient text *Atharva Veda*, ginseng causes a man to exhale a fire-like heat.

According to most Asian physicians, ginseng works as an aphrodisiac for two reasons. First, it helps create a surge of vitality. Second—and more important—it revives and invigorates the body as a whole. This helps ensure an adequate supply of hormones and a well-functioning reproductive system.

## Asian, American, and Siberian Ginseng

There are three different types of ginseng: the Asian variety (*Panax ginseng*), American ginseng (*Panax quinquefolius*), and Siberian ginseng (*Eleutherococcus senticosus*). Asian ginseng usually comes from China or Korea. In North America, wild ginseng grows in rich, cool woods from Maine to Georgia and west to Oklahoma and Minnesota. Siberian ginseng is not true ginseng, but it has many of the properties of ginseng and is used in the same ways.

It is the "true" ginsengs, Asian and American, that became known as aphrodisiacs. Animal studies tend to confirm that reputation. Male rats fed Asian ginseng became far more sexually active. Studies of ginseng-fed rabbits, bulls, and rats indicate that ginseng encourages growth of the gonads and improves the potency of sperm in males.

## An Adaptogen

Ginseng is not used as a treatment for specific illnesses. Rather, it is an overall health builder and revitalizer. Ginseng is what is known as an "adaptogen"—that is, it has the ability to adapt itself to individual requirements. It acts to normalize and balance the body's functions for each individual who uses it. For example, ginseng contains substances that enable it to adapt itself to the hormonal needs of women going through menopause. Ginseng is believed to increase estrogen levels in women and is thus helpful in treating menopausal symptoms such as hot flashes.

Other uses of ginseng: To heal the nervous system, regulate blood pressure, control cholesterol, regulate blood sugar and body weight, overcome fatigue, prevent atherosclerosis, treat anemia.

Very large doses of ginseng may cause insomnia or anxiety.

Ginseng should not be used where there is high fever or hypertension because it will aggravate these conditions.

Ginseng should not be used if there is edema or if there are kidney problems because ginseng is an antidiuretic. It will aggravate these conditions.

Ginseng is a blood thinner and should not be used if you are taking anticoagulant drugs or aspirin.

## *Licorice (Glycyrrhiza glabra)*

Licorice tones and stimulates the female sex glands. Its root has been an important herb in Chinese medicine for over five thousand years. Like ginkgo and ginseng, licorice is used to treat a wide variety of ailments. The energy-enhancing properties of licorice can make for a more active sex life.

Licorice is especially beneficial for those who suffer from adrenal gland exhaustion. The adrenal glands sit on top of the kidneys. They are stimulated by stress (both psychological and physical) and produce the hormones adrenalin and noradrenalin in response to it. Adrenalin pours sugar into the blood for the energy we need to deal with a crisis. It raises blood pressure and directs blood to the muscles and brain to give us the added strength and brain power to deal with the stress. Noradrenalin acts in a similar way except that it lowers the heart rate.

When the body, mind, or emotions are subjected to prolonged stress, the adrenals become exhausted. Symptoms of adrenal exhaustion are far from conducive to sex. They include chronic fatigue, irritability, weakness, inability to concentrate, indigestion, and depression.

Licorice root is very high in natural starches and sugars, which are quickly converted to energy, primarily through the liver and adrenal glands. Licorice rests and strengthens the adrenals. This enables the body to recover from exhaustion.

Another important use of licorice root is to treat problems of the female reproductive system. Licorice helps regulate the menstrual cycle because it contains significant amounts of plant estrogens. It is included in many herbal preparations aimed at treating symptoms of menopause, as most of these symptoms are caused by lowered estrogen levels.

Other uses of licorice: To expel mucus from the respiratory tract, purify the blood and promote circulation, relieve stomach ulcers, and treat bladder and kidney ailments.

Do not use licorice if you have high blood pressure, except under medical supervision. Large doses will increase blood pressure.

### *Oats* (*Avena sativa*)

Recently, oats have been publicized as a sex booster. Will taking an oat supplement help you to "feel your oats"? So far there is no scientific evidence to suggest this will happen. However, oats have a mildly stimulating effect, and users claim they are a sex tonic and aphrodisiac.

According to folklore, the discovery of the aphrodisiacal properties of oats was made by a Chinese grain farmer who raised koi (large carp) as a hobby. He kept the fish food in a bag in the barn and asked his son to feed the fish each day before he went to school. The boy did so. When the bag was empty, he told his father he needed more food. The father was surprised the food was gone so quickly. When he went to the barn to check, he discovered that his son had taken food from the wrong bag. He had fed the fish green oats.

The farmer rushed to the pond, expecting to find all his precious koi dead. Instead, hundreds of baby fish were swimming in the pond. Something in the oats had caused the fish to breed more aggressively. Thus was sown the reputation of wild oats as an aphrodisiac.

Other uses of oats: To strengthen the nervous system, treat exhaustion and depression, and improve digestion.

### Sarsaparilla *(Smilax officinalis)*

Today sarsaparilla is most commonly known as a carbonated drink and a flavoring agent in root beer. But to Native Americans, sarsaparilla was an aphrodisiac, male tonic, and treatment for urinary problems. Native to Central America, sarsaparilla was brought to Europe in the sixteenth century. At first it was used to treat syphilis, but it soon became known as a tonic for male potency.

Because sarsaparilla contains plant steroid-like components (saponin glycosides), it is currently included in body-building formulas to increase muscle mass. There is no evidence, however, to back up the claim that saponins increase muscle mass as steroids do.

Although some herbalists claim that sarsaparilla contains male hormones, chemical analysis does not indicate this. Its saponins, however, do stimulate the body's metabolism. They promote urination and sweating and help expel mucus from the lungs. Hence sarsaparilla is known as a body purifier and as a tonic for the urinary tract.

Other uses of sarsaparilla: To treat skin eruptions, ringworm, rheumatism, and gout.

### Saw Palmetto *(Serenoa serrulata)*

One of the best herbs for the prostate, saw palmetto is a shrub commonly found along the southeast coast of North America. It is a fan-shaped herb that looks like a type of palm. The red-brown berries of saw palmetto were eaten by Native American men to increase sexual vigor, and by women to firm the breasts. The usual dosage was four to five berries a day.

Prostatitis (inflammation of the prostate) is a painful condition that can inhibit sexual activity. In herbal preparations for the prostate, saw palmetto is often combined with an extract made from *pygeum africanum,* an evergreen tree native to Africa and Madagascar. Through its diuretic actions the extract relieves some of the pain of prostatitis. Saw palmetto reduces inflammation in the prostate tissues and helps reduce cholesterol deposits in the prostate.

Other uses of saw palmetto: To treat asthma, bronchitis, low libido, menstrual irregularities, prostate enlargement, sinus and respiratory problems, and sterility.

### Schisandra *(Schisandra chinesis)*

Schisandra, or schizandra, is an herb highly prized in China. It was known to be a favorite among Chinese emperors. Chinese men use it as a general tonic and sex stimulant; women use it as a sex stimulant and preserver of beauty. Schisandra is also claimed to be an antidepressant.

Like ginseng and ginkgo, schisandra is an adaptogen used to combat fatigue and stress and to increase stamina. In northern China some tribes took dried schisandra berries on hunting trips to help them maintain energy and strength, especially during the winter.

Recent research indicates that schisandra may well increase aerobic activity and stamina. When polo horses were fed an extract of schisandra berries they showed improved aerobic activity and better responses to stress. During exercise their heart rate did not increase as much, and their breathing rate returned to normal more quickly.

Other uses of schisandra: To beautify the skin, strength the entire body, and improve mental functioning and memory.

### St. John's Wort *(Hypericum perforatum)*

St. John's wort has long been used as a treatment for depression, anxiety, and insomnia—all enemies of a healthy sex drive. The yellow flowers and tops of the plants have been used for centuries in Europe to treat many types of nervous conditions. It is taken either as a tea or in an olive oil extract.

Researchers in Germany studied St. John's wort for decades, and German regulators have approved prescribing the herb to elevate mood and treat depression. A study reported in the *British Medical Journal* in August, 1996, concluded that extracts of St. John's wort were effective for the treatment of mild to moderately severe depressive disorders. They were just as effective as standard prescription antidepressants, with far fewer side effects.

Scientific interest in St. John's wort has increased recently because of its potential as an antivirus agent against AIDS. When mice infected with HIV-like viruses were given extracts of St. John's wort, the progress of the viruses was halted. Testing was then done on human patients with the HIV virus and AIDS. Results are inconclusive, though significant improvement was reported in some patients.

St. John's wort grows wild in the meadows of Europe. In the United States it is available in health food stores and from herb suppliers, and comes in liquid, capsule, and dried form.

Other uses of St. John's wort: To treat asthma, anemia, diarrhea, colic, and coughs. Externally, an oil tincture is applied to treat tumors, swollen breasts, sciatic pain, ulcers, and wounds.

If you have fair skin, avoid exposure to strong sunlight and ultraviolet light while taking St. John's wort. Some photosensitivity has been reported.

St. John's wort contains a type of antidepressant called an MAO inhibitor. The herb (and prescription MAO inhibitors) should not be taken with foods rich in tyramine (e.g., cheese, liver, red wine). Interaction with tyramine causes severe headaches and hazardously high blood pressure. Similarly, tyrosine interacts with MAO inhibitors to increase blood pressure. Tyrosine supplements should not be taken with St. John's wort.

Narcotics, amphetamines, alcoholic beverages, and over-the-counter cold and flu remedies can interact with MAO inhibitors to increase blood pressure. Thus they should not be taken with St. John's wort.

St. John's wort probably should not be used during pregnancy or lactation.

### Vitex  (*Vitex agnus-castus*)

Vitex is made from the fruit of a shrub that is commonly known as the chaste tree. Native to Asia, the chaste tree is now found throughout Europe and the southern United States. The *castus* part of its botanical name, meaning "chaste" in Greek, stems from the belief that the berries *lowered* sex drive. Medieval priests and nuns drank vitex syrup to maintain chastity. Arabs and Egyptians, on the other hand, believed the berries were a powerful aphrodisiac.

Although neither group was entirely right, the Arabs and Egyptians were closer to the truth. While vitex is not a fast-acting aphrodisiac, it helps normalize the reproductive system. Research in Germany indicates that vitex can balance the production of sex hormones. Vitex works by stimulating the pituitary gland to secrete the luteinizing hormone, which helps control the functioning of the sex organs.

Vitex has long been known as a remedy for women's problems. It is an herb used by European women for its positive effects on the reproductive system, especially during and after pregnancy. It is said to increase the flow of breast milk.

Other uses of vitex: To regain strength after overindulgence.

### Wild Yam  (*Dioscirea villosa*)

Although wild yam is used to manufacture synthetic DHEA and progesterone, there is no evidence that eating wild yam will stimulate the body's own production of those two hormones. Wild yam is different from the cultivated yam or sweet potato. You probably would not enjoy eating wild yam.

# ❧ USING HERBS EFFECTIVELY AND SAFELY

Herbal preparations are available in many forms from health food stores, herb stores, and mail-order sources. Herb seeds and plants are also available for those who want to grow their own. Gathering herbs in the wild can be hazardous unless you are well versed in botany, since some herbs have toxic look-alikes. Other herbs are toxic in their raw form, but medicinal when dried or cooked. Whatever your source of herbs, you will need to know how to use them. Here is a short summary of different ways herbs are prepared and used.

# ❧ HERBAL PREPARATIONS

## *Capsules and Pills*
Herbs are often sold in capsule or pill form for people who do not care for their taste or smell. Capsules should be stored in a cool, dark place. Some need to be refrigerated (these are stored in refrigerated cases in stores, and the label contains a notice about keeping them refrigerated). Pills are not as apt to stick together as capsules and may be better for traveling, especially in a warm car. Capsules, on the other hand, are assimilated more quickly and completely by the body.

Vegetarians may not want to take capsules made from gelatin, an animal product. Vegetable-based capsules are available, including ones that you fill yourself.

If capsules are taken between meals they should be taken with at least half a cup of water. They can be rubbed with a little water or vegetable oil if they are difficult to swallow.

## *Herbal Tea*
Herbs with a mild or pleasant flavor are often used in tea form. Health food stores carry a wide assortment of herbal

teas that have already been dried, cut, and sifted for use. If you make tea with fresh herbs, first rub them between your hands or grind them with a mortar and pestle. Tea is brewed either by infusion or decoction.

### *Infusion*
What we usually think of as tea is an infusion. The herbs themselves are not boiled, but steeped. To make an infusion:

- Use about 1 ounce of dried herbs, or 2 ounces of fresh herbs, to a pint of water.
- Put the herbs in a container that can be tightly closed.
- Boil the water in a nonmetal or stainless steel pot. Use distilled water or spring water if possible.
- When the water comes to a rolling boil, pour it over the herb.
- Cover the container tightly and let it stand about twenty minutes.
- Strain it and drink the clear tea.

An infusion can also be made without boiling the water. Simply put the herb in a glass jar, add water, and cover it tightly. Put the jar in the sun for a few hours. The result is called sun tea.

### *Decoction*
Decoctions, usually made from roots or bark, are used to extract the deeper essences of the herb. The herb is simmered in water for about an hour until half the water has evaporated. Most herbs are simmered uncovered, but some that contain important oils (such as cinnamon, burdock, and valerian) are simmered in a covered pot.

Both infusions and decoctions should be used within 24 to 72 hours, before they start to sour or spoil. Refrigerate unused tea.

## Tincture

A tincture is a concentrated extract of an herb, usually in an alcohol base. Because alcohol is a preservative, tinctures can be kept for a long period of time. Tinctures are convenient because they can be carried around easily and can be swallowed with just a small amount of water. Or they can be added to juices or placed under the tongue. Tinctures are readily absorbed by the body and begin to work quickly. Some herbs are customarily taken in tinctures because they are not soluble in water and thus cannot be consumed as tea.

For those who do not wish to use alcohol, the tincture dose can be stirred in a small amount of boiling water to evaporate the alcohol.

To make a tincture, follow these steps:

- Combine 4 ounces of the powdered herb with 1 pint of alcohol (e.g., gin, brandy, rum, vodka) or apple cider vinegar.

- Keep the mixture in a tightly covered jar or bottle and let it stand for two weeks. Shake it twice a day.

- Let the herb settle to the bottom and pour the tincture into a dark glass bottle, straining the liquid through a filter or piece of muslin.

- If you wish, seal the top with melted wax.

The final concentration of alcohol should be at least 30 percent. To figure out the concentration of alcohol, divide the proof number of the alcohol you used in half. For example, if you used 80 proof liquor, the alcohol content would be 40 percent. Tinctures can be diluted by mixing them with water.

## Electuary

An electuary is a powdered herb mixed with honey, peanut butter, maple syrup, or slippery elm to form a paste, and then rolled into a ball. This is a good method to use with strong or unpleasant-tasting herbs. Measure the powdered herb first, then add the sweetener.

## ๑ HOW TO OBTAIN HERBS SAFELY

"Natural" does not always mean safe. The poison in some plants is more deadly than a cobra's. And some beneficial members of the plant kingdom have poisonous look-alikes. As the saying goes, "There are old mushroom hunters. And there are bold mushroom hunters. But there are no old, bold mushroom hunters."

Unless you are well educated in plant lore, it is safer to obtain your herbal supplies in a health food store or pharmacy rather than gather them yourself in the wild.


## ๑ SHOULD YOU GROW YOUR OWN?

If you grow your own herbs, be careful about experimenting with unknown varieties. According to the Food and Drug Administration, most of the problems with toxicity from herbs have been with people who grow their own. The problem stems from the fact that they have not had the training and experience in using herbs that is passed down traditionally from generation to generation in other countries.

Another problem of do-it-yourselfers is dosage. The potency of an herbal preparation can vary depending on how it is prepared and even on the individual plants from which it is made. For some herbs the difference between a therapeutic dose and a toxic dose is slight. Without extensive training in the traditional methods of preparing and using herbs, it is easy to overdose.

Are commercial herbal preparations safer than homemade ones? Most manufacturers of herbal products do not include dangerous herbs in their products. But it never hurts to be informed—and to read labels.

# ❧ HERBS THAT MAY CAUSE PROBLEMS

The FDA lists nine herbs that have the potential for causing serious health problems, including kidney failure and stroke. They are:

- Chaparral
- Comfrey
- Germander
- Jin bu huan
- Lobelia
- Magnolia
- Ma huang
- Stephania
- Yohimbe

# ❧ DANGEROUS HERBAL APHRODISIACS

A few so-called aphrodisiacs can be dangerous if not used under the guidance of a physician. One, Spanish fly, can be fatal. Even if a substance is not toxic, there is always the possibility that you will be allergic to it, or that by combining it with other ingredients you may have adverse reactions.

## *Spanish Fly*
Beware of any aphrodisiac preparation that contains cantharidin. This is a substance made from the powdered remains of the Mediterranean cantharis beetle *(Cantharis vesicatoria)*, more commonly known as "Spanish fly." Spanish fly is reputed to be an aphrodisiac because it stimulates the penis and vagina. It works by severely irritating (and even blistering) the mucous membrane of the genitourinary tract.

It inflames the lining of the bladder and urethra. In men, this causes a painful, prolonged erection, and in women, an engorged clitoris. It can also inflame the kidneys and lining of the intestines and create intense urinary burning, abdominal pain, nausea, diarrhea, and the urge to urinate.

Spanish fly is classified as a Class 1 poison by the US government. A few milligrams can cause kidney damage or failure, and 30 mg or more may be fatal. Spanish fly has caused fatal comas. It is an extremely dangerous substance.

### *Ma Huang or Ephedra* (*Ephedra sinica*)

For centuries, Chinese herbalists have used ma huang (also called ephedra) to treat such conditions as asthma and upper respiratory infection. Today, however, people are taking this herb for a "legal high," a substitute for illegal recreational drugs such as Ecstasy and methamphetamine, which are used to heighten sexual feelings. Even though ma huang is currently legal, concern is growing that it can cause such adverse reactions as irregular heartbeat, heart attack, stroke, seizures, psychosis, and even death by cardiac arrest.

Ephedra formulas have been marketed under such brand names as Herbal Ecstasy, Cloud 9, and Ultimate Xphoria. The FDA has never tested or approved any herbal ephedra compound. In fact, the FDA does not test or approve herbal products.

Ephedra compounds are also sold to increase energy and weight loss. In 1995 the FDA received more than 100 reports of injuries and adverse reactions from one such formula, *Nature's Nutrition Formula 1.* The manufacturers of another ephedra product that was promoted as a muscle builder were named in a wrongful-death suit of a seventeen-year-old boy who died as a result of using the product.

### *Jimson Weed, or Thorn Apple*

Jimson weed, like ma huang, supposedly boosts the sex drive by producing a "high." This high, however, comes at a high price. Jimson weed can be fatal. The word "jimson" is a corruption of "Jamestown." It was in Jamestown, Virginia is 1676 that the first deaths from eating the plant were recorded.

Jimson is an intoxicating plant. It is also highly toxic. In the 1800s it was used before surgery as a narcotic and pain reliever. Today it is not sold in stores or used in herbal preparations. Unfortunately, this does not stop foolish people from searching for it in the wild. (Even handling the plant can cause swollen eyelids.) In 1994 more than a dozen young people in New York and Connecticut were hospitalized after experimenting with jimson weed. More recently two Texas teenagers died as a result of eating jimson weed for its intoxicating effects.

### Mandrake

Mandrake is a forked root that became known as an aphrodisiac because, like ginseng, it resembles the human form. Unlike ginseng, however, mandrake can be dangerous. It is easy to overdose on mandrake and be poisoned by this member of the deadly nightshade family.

There are two varieties of mandrake, the spring and the fall. Both are native to the Mediterranean and Himalayan regions, especially to Greece. In spite of its putrid odor, people have sought out this dangerous root for centuries. Considered "magical," mandrake was used not only as an aphrodisiac but as a charm for pregnancy, invulnerability, and for discovering treasure. In medieval times it was administered as a narcotic before surgery.

### Marijuana (Cannabis sativa)

Marijuana—especially the female plant—is narcotic. At first it is exhilarating and an aphrodisiac, but after a while it acts as a sedative. There is evidence that heavy use of marijuana can lead to temporary sterility.

Marijuana diminishes male potency in the same way as alcohol—by decreasing levels of the male hormone testosterone. Testosterone decreases proportionately to the amount of marijuana smoked. When testosterone levels go down, a man's sex drive decreases.

What about women? Is the female sex drive also lowered by smoking pot? It can be. Women produce testosterone, too, just as men produce small amounts of female hormones. In women, testosterone is produced by the ovaries and the adrenal glands. A drop in a woman's testosterone level may diminish her sex drive. For some women it can also result in difficulty in achieving an orgasm.

(See pp. 169–170 for more information on how street drugs affect sexuality.)

### Poison Nut (Strychnos nux vomica)
True to its name, poison nut can be toxic. It can also be therapeutic. It depends on the dosage—and the difference between a therapeutic and toxic dose is slight. The sexually stimulating ingredient in poison nut is strychnine, a deadly poison. This does not seem to deter foolhardy aphrodisiac seekers, who use strychnine as a sexual stimulant.

## CHAPTER FOUR

## *Pheromones as Aphrodisiacs*

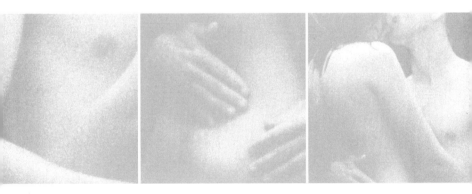

*S*mell is perhaps the oldest and most primitive of our five senses. Yet of all our senses, we know the least about it. We are only beginning to discover the power of smell and how it is linked to sex. What we have found out so far is startling.

Until recently, scientists were not much interested in the sense of smell. They preferred to spend their time investigating the "higher" senses of sight and hearing. Any suggestion that smell might be linked to sex, as it is with animals, was dismissed or ignored. In part, this attitude was a carryover from Victorian times, when bodily odors—especially sexual ones—were considered unsavory. But now there is an explosion of research on how the sense of smell and sex are linked. What caused this intense interest? It began with the discovery of a tiny organ in the human nose that senses substances called pheromones.

In the animal world, smell is a powerful sexual stimulant. (Anyone who has had a dog or cat "in heat" can attest to that!) With animals it is love at first smell. One whiff of a receptive female drives males to a frenzy. Physical beauty and visual cues count for nothing. It is her scent that is irresistible. It draws males on with an overpowering urge to mate and ensures that she will reproduce, that the species will continue. For most mammals, smell is the only aphrodisiac.

With humans it is different. Our intellect and emotions play a major role in finding a mate, as do our senses of sight and hearing. Still, we share most of our genes with our closest animal relatives, the higher primates. Isn't it possible that nature made us, too, susceptible to the pull of sexual scents?

For years researchers largely ignored the possibility that we might be like other animals in this regard. Humans reportedly experience love at first sight. Love at first smell? Not likely. Besides, what if it were true? Suppose chemical messages from another individual could influence our behavior without our even being aware of it. We could become unwitting victims of a kind of biochemical brainwashing. The prospect is disturbing, to say the least. After all, we are creatures of free will—aren't we?

## ❧ DISCOVERY OF PHEROMONES

In the early 1980s the picture began to change. Two separate groups of researchers presented evidence that, like animals, we have a special organ in our nose that detects chemical signals. This organ is called the VNO (vomeronasal organ). Its entrance is in the nostrils through two tiny slits almost invisible to the naked eye.

In animals the VNO detects chemical messages from other animals of the same species. These messages are called *pheromones* (from the Greek *pherein*, "to carry," and *hormon*, "to excite"). Pheromones are like airborne hormones. As their name implies, they excite.

The discovery of a human VNO raised important questions: Do humans produce pheromones? Are humans affected by pheromones? If so, how? Research on human pheromones began in earnest.

Sometimes an important discovery is made by accident. Such was the case with human pheromones. In the 1970s Dr. David Berliner was Professor of Anatomy at the University of Utah. As part of his research on the chemistry of the skin, he scraped skin cells from used plaster casts of skiers who had broken bones on the Utah slopes. He made extracts from the cells and put them in open vials in the laboratory.

A strange thing happened. The hectic lab quieted down. The usual bickering stopped and lab workers became cheerful, cordial. They even lunched together and played bridge. When Berliner capped the vials, the lab reverted to its customary noisy discord. This happened more than once. It seemed that whenever Berliner kept the vials open, people (including him) felt better. They became warmer, friendlier, more open. When

Berliner closed the vials, discord returned to the lab. Something rising from the extracts seemed to change feelings and behavior. Yet the extracts had no odor. Whatever was occurring, it was not happening through the sense of smell. Intrigued and puzzled, Berliner froze the extracts for future research.

When Berliner heard about the discovery of the human VNO, he suspected that the active substances in his vials might be human pheromones. In 1989 he developed two synthetic compounds based on his extracts of male and female skin cells. He enlisted the help of Dr. Luis Monti-Bloch to test their effect on the human VNO. Monti-Bloch devised an apparatus to measure electrical impulses in the VNO though a probe as fine as a hair. Using a microspritzer, he puffed four kinds of substances to the VNOs of volunteers: (1) plain air; (2) Berliner's two compounds; (3) a solution with no odor and no pheromones; (4) a fragrant clove essence mixture with no pheromones. He used a double-blind procedure, meaning that neither the subject nor clinician knew which substance was being released into the nose.

The subjects' VNOs reacted *only* to Berliner's extracts. Even more startling—the VNOs of male subjects reacted only to female extracts; the VNOs of female subjects reacted only to male extracts.

Monti-Bloch repeated the experiment, this time attaching the probe to olfactory ("smell") nerves in the nose. These nerves reacted only to the substance with an odor, the essence of cloves. The fact that Berliner's compounds were detected by the VNO, but not by smell, indicated that they were probably human pheromones. The fact that their effect was gender specific indicated that they were probably sex pheromones.

Berliner's findings raised intriguing questions. Are human sex pheromones aphrodisiacs? Do they affect the body? behavior? emotions? Do they affect men and women differently?

As the story of pheromones unfolds, it promises to challenge many of our beliefs about human sexuality. The following is a summary of what researchers have learned thus far.

# ❧ HOW PHEROMONES WORK

We begin making pheromones at puberty and continue at a fairly steady rate until about age fifty for women and seventy for men. Pheromone production then begins to decline along with declining levels of sex hormones.

Most pheromones are produced in special sweat glands (apocrine glands) that are attached to hair follicles. Apocrine glands are heavily concentrated in areas where hair appears in puberty: the underarms, genital and anal areas, chest, lower abdomen, and areas surrounding the nipples and navel.

Hairs trap gland secretions next to the skin, where bacteria begin to decompose them. During the decomposition process, pheromones are released.

Pheromones are released into the air in the sweat that evaporates from our skin and in the approximately forty million skin cells we shed each day. Once airborne, our pheromone messages can be conveniently "read" by any passing human who happens to inhale them. Pheromones are also present in saliva, and from the saliva they pass into the breath.

## Male and Female Scents

As bacteria break down glandular secretions, their action produces odors as well as pheromones. Male pheromones are accompanied by a musky odor which forms part of the male scent. Most men also have special strains of odor-producing skin bacteria that contribute to the male odor. Some women have the bacteria, too, but their levels of the female hormone estrogen prevent them from having a strong male odor.

The scent of a woman has been described as sweet and subtle. It is associated with pheromones derived from the female hormones estrogen and progesterone. A woman's odor fluctuates with hormone levels during the monthly cycle. It is less intense than that of a man. Pheromone-connected odors vary from person to person because of varying levels of hormones, differing biochemistry, and genetics. For each of us, pheromone-connected odors are a major component of our "smellprint."

## Smellprints

Each of us has a smellprint, an individual pheromone/odor signature as unique as our fingerprints. Slight, distinguishing odor differences are caused by our gender, genes, environment, and lifestyle. Because our smellprint has a pheromone base, it is detected by the VNO and cannot be camouflaged with odors—no matter how sensuous or distracting. Perfumes, colognes, deodorants notwithstanding, phero-mones win out. The nose knows.

When we meet, we unknowingly exchange pheromone signatures. Perceived unconsciously, they nevertheless reveal much. What they say helps determine our reaction to the other person. They are part of the chemistry that draws two people together, part of the reason two strangers can meet and instantly feel as if they have known each other all their lives.

## Are Pheromones Aphrodisiacs?

According to Dr. David Berliner, human sex pheromones are not technically aphrodisiacs in that they do not directly stimulate sexual activity. Rather, they enhance sensuality and improve mood. Berliner patented synthetic pheromones and incorporated them in fragrances for men and women, which are sold under the brand name *Realm*. *Realm* promotional material takes care to dispel the notion that pheromones are aphrodisiacs. Rather, it says that the scents were developed to benefit the *person who wears them.*

Wearers have reported that the scents make them feel warm, comfortable, self-confident, and more at ease. They also feel more attractive, romantic, and alluring.

Most would agree with Berliner that pheromones are not irresistible sexual lures. This is not to say, however, that they do not affect humans sexually. Research has turned up some intriguing data on exactly what pheromones can do.

### Male Pheromones

*Effects on Women*

- Regular exposure to male pheromones helps normalize the menstrual cycle. It makes it shorter and more regular.
- Each month, a woman's susceptibility to male pheromones peaks at the time of ovulation, when she is most fertile.
- Exposure to male pheromones in musk can cause women to ovulate more readily and become more easily aroused.
- Regular exposure to male pheromones accelerates the beginning of puberty for girls.

*Effects on Men*

- Among animals, the whiff of male pheromones—especially androstenone—makes other males aggressive. In humans, androstenone is a strong presence in male sweat. Could this help explain aggressive behavior of males who congregate—and sweat—together?
- James Vaughn Kohl and Robert T. Francoeur, authors of *The Scent of Eros*, note that there is speculation about this connection between male aggression and the smell of male sweat. They cite as examples hostile graffiti in men's restrooms, aggressive behavior of men in large groups and on the hockey rink, basketball court, or football field.
- Researchers at Birmingham University sprayed a chair in an office waiting room with a mist containing the male pheromone androstenone, which has a urine-like smell. Men avoided sitting in the chair, especially when

androstenone was applied in heavier doses. (Women were attracted to the chair.)

- Exposure to androstenone may stir erotic memories or sexual desire.

## Female Pheromones

### Effects on Men

- Regular contact with women reportedly makes the beard grow more rapidly. The presence of female pheromones can stimulate production of male hormones. This, in turn, stimulates beard growth.

- There is anecdotal evidence from sexual folklore that the sweat and vaginal secretions of a woman are aphrodisiacs, but this has not been scientifically proven. (Both sweat and vaginal secretions contain female pheromones.)

### Effects on Women

- When women live with other women they tend to have their menstrual period at about the same time. This synchronization is caused by "messages" from female pheromones transmitted in sweat. Often their menstrual cycles become synchronized with that of the dominant woman in the group.

- Long-term exposure to female pheromones may increase sexual desire among women. In one double-blind study, young women were exposed either to female pheromones or to a placebo. After fourteen weeks, the percentage of women having sex on a weekly basis increased from 11 percent to 73 percent for women receiving the pheromones. It remained the same for those who received the placebo.

# ❧ USING PHEROMONES TO ENHANCE SEX

Typically, love potions in folklore contain body secretions. Whether it be urine, sweat, semen, or menstrual blood, the pheromone-rich substance is promised to create instant lust or everlasting fidelity in the unsuspecting victim.

The use of love potions continues today. In rural areas of Brazil women serve an intended lover coffee filtered though their unlaundered underwear. In New Guinea a man will waft a handkerchief suffused with underarm sweat under the nose of the woman he desires.

Pheromones are fascinating, but aside from providing provocative conversation for cocktail parties, what can pheromone savvy do for you and your sex life?

- *It can help you understand the chemistry of sexual attraction*—why you can be strangely attracted to a certain someone, even when your friends tell you, "I don't know what you see in him (or her)."

- *It makes you aware of society's attempts to suppress your pheromones*—for example, by persuading you to deodorize yourself or to wear restrictive clothing that traps your pheromones. Rather than being unknowingly manipulated in this way, you will be able to decide for yourself whether you wish to follow such restrictions.

- *It makes you an informed consumer, less likely to succumb to extravagant advertising claims for pheromone-based products.* Knowledge of what human pheromones can and can't do will help you think twice before putting out money for a product that claims its pheromone content will make you instantly irresistible to any prospect within whiffing distance or that it will inflate your sex drive to enviable proportions.

Pheromones are subliminal persuaders, designed by nature to ensure that we attract and choose a biologically suitable mate. There are a number of ways you can use pheromone knowledge to enhance this process.

### Using Armpit Allure

The armpit is one of the most alluring areas of the human body because of its concentration of pheromone-producing apocrine glands and because of underarm hair—which in itself is a sexual attractant. The armpit figures prominently in courtship behavior and the exchange of pheromones. Take slow dancing, for example. Partners stand face-to-face with their arms partially raised, allowing clouds of pheromones to escape from their armpits.

To take full advantage of pheromone power, expose your armpits. Lift your arms away from your sides and liberate your pheromones. Holding your arms close to your body effectively suppresses pheromone distribution, just as a male dog suppresses his pheromones by tucking his tail between his legs and holding it tightly against his body to avoid irritating a more aggressive male.

### Avoiding the Clothing Trap

At times when you want your pheromones to be released into the air, avoid clothing that traps them, for example, body-hugging clothing made of Lycra™ or any other tightly woven fabric.

Cultural and religious customs that require covering the head may not consciously have been instituted to discourage intimacy by hindering pheromone release, but that is the result. Wearing a veil, scarf, turban, or hat effectively inhibits the free release of pheromones from the hair, which is an especially abundant source.

### To Shave, or Not to Shave?

Together the skin, glands, bacteria, and hair create a working pheromone factory. What happens when a woman shaves her underarms and legs? Theoretically, what she gains in aesthetics she may lose in pheromones, at least temporarily. Underarm hair helps trap body secretions and increases skin warmth for pheromone evaporation.

## No Sweat?

When Napoleon asked Josephine not to bathe for three days (see p. 72), he was not alone in his aromatic preferences. The "sweat is sensual" school continues to have its advocates, despite the best efforts of all those who seek to deodorize us as a species. Considering what we know about pheromones, maybe we should throw out our deodorants, aftershaves, perfumes, and colognes and instead just work up a good sweat.

It is not unusual to love the sweaty scent of a lover, because that sweat carries the lover's smellprint. It is unique, and immediately recalls the lover's physical presence in a way that even a photograph cannot. That is why a woman may wear her lover's T-shirt, and why people find themselves sleeping on the other side of the bed when their lover is gone. The lingering smellprint is a comforting reminder of the lover's physical presence.

## No Smell?

Suppose the issue is not "to smell or not to smell," but that you can't smell—either temporarily, because of a cold, or permanently (a condition called anosmia). The good news is that although you cannot smell odors, you can still perceive pheromones through your VNO.

## Don't Fight Your Pheromones

If the "chemistry isn't right" in a romance, consider that your pheromones might be trying to tell you something. Perhaps your partner's immune system is too similar to yours. Based on animal studies, it appears that we unconsciously "read" a prospective lover's pheromones to help us find a mate with a compatible immunotype (someone whose genes carry immunities we do not have). Given a choice of mates, rats use smell to find a mate with a different immunotype. In fact, they choose the one who is *most* different. Opposites attract. It is nature's way of distributing genes—and immunities—throughout a species.

## Too Good to Be True?

When human pheromones hit the news, they made a big splash in the media. Articles about pheromones appeared in major newspapers and magazines, and they were discussed on radio and TV talk shows. Advertisements and infomercials for products containing pheromones were quick to follow, as well as numerous offerings on the Internet. As a result, you can supplement your own pheromones with spray-on, rub-on, or splash-on versions that will work sexual magic—if the products live up to their extravagant advertising claims. For example: *Pheromones attract, compel, make you irresistible...Others will be drawn to you without knowing why...Pheromones give you the secret advantage over other men (women).*

Your knowledge of pheromones will help you evaluate such claims. If you do decide to try a pheromone product, you will be doing it with your eyes open. Keep in mind, though, that there is such a thing as a placebo effect. You often get what you expect. As the old adage advises, "If it sounds too good to be true, it probably is."

# CHAPTER FIVE

*Aromas as Aphrodisiacs*

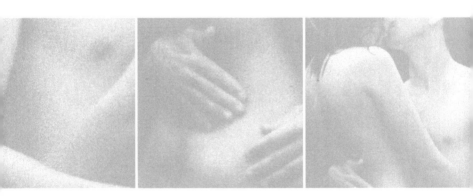

$S$o far we have been concerned with the auxiliary sense of smell and the sexual messages carried by pheromones. What about the primary sense of smell? Can scents and odors arouse us sexually? Can they set the mood for romance? Absolutely. For proof, we need look no further than the multi-billion-dollar perfume industry. But there is scientific proof as well. It is based on how smell receptors in the nose connect to the brain.

## ❧ WHY AROMAS AROUSE US

Of the five senses, only the sense of smell bypasses the cerebral cortex—the conscious "thinking" part of our brain. Smell receptors in the nose are directly wired to the limbic center, the part of the brain that controls our sex drive, emotions, and sensual memories. Thus a smell can arouse us, trigger an emotion, or evoke a memory, and our conscious mind cannot control our response.

For example, we may get a whiff of sandalwood, a scent always worn by someone we dislike. Instantly—against our will—we are reminded of him/her. And the memory brings with it strong emotions associated with that person. Suddenly we feel angry, annoyed, or depressed without knowing why. We take an immediate, unexplainable dislike to the person who innocently wears the offending fragrance. That odor is forever connected with negative emotions in our limbic brain.

In a long-term relationship, a mate's scent is internalized and can become a critical factor in the way people positively relate to one another. Anitra Earle, "The Perfume Detective," receives some two thousand pleas a year asking her to find a long-loved, but discontinued fragrance. Earle says, "I get long letters that say things like, '*If you can find this perfume you can save my marriage.*' Sometimes they're kidding—but sometimes they mean it."

## ☙ JOSEPHINE'S REVENGE!

Fragrances definitely have personalities—qualities as diverse and many-faceted as their wearers. Keeping this in mind, many people adopt a signature scent—a fragrance that will always be associated with them. This can prove useful. A drop of fragrance on a love letter can increase its impact. On the other hand, if revenge is on your mind, take a lesson from Napoleon's Josephine.

Napoleon preferred his woman with a gamy "three days unwashed" odor. He is said to have written Josephine, "*Je reviens en trois jours, ne te lave pas!*" (I will return in three days. Do not bathe!) Those oft-quoted words inspired the perfume *Je Reviens*, produced by the couture House of Worth.

Josephine, however, loved musk and used it liberally; it became her signature scent. When Napoleon eventually rejected her, she poured musk all over the imperial bedroom, over all the wooden surfaces and into the carpeting to make sure he would never forget her. Her revenge was sweet and lasting. (The scent of musk is extremely tenacious!)

## ☙ AROMATHERAPY

Aromatherapy promises to reveal the powers of *phyto* (plant) chemicals and show us how to use the aromatic oils of plants for many purposes:
- To stimulate or soothe the body
- To arouse or quiet the emotions
- To elevate mood
- To alter mental states
- To improve psychic and spiritual awareness
- To create whatever aromatic ambiance we desire

It is beyond the scope of this book to provide a comprehensive discussion of aromatherapy. Fortunately, there are many fine books available on the subject. Suffice it to say that like herbs, aromas and aromatic plant oils can enhance sex in two ways:

- By directly stimulating the body
- By giving rise to emotions that are conducive to lovemaking

The section that follows describes the first group, erotic scents, in some detail. After that are two charts that list aromatic oils used to enhance mood and the emotions.

Essential oils are usually used as inhalants, or they are mixed with base oils (such as grapeseed or almond), and massaged on the skin.

Several cautions:

- Never put an essential oil near your eyes.
- Always dilute an oil before applying it to your body as it may severely irritate the skin.
- If you are pregnant or if you have sensitive skin or allergies, research an oil carefully before you decide to try it.
- Since some essential oils deteriorate latex, they should not be used to lubricate condoms. Essential oils may also irritate the mucous membranes.

## ✺ EROTIC SCENTS TO STIMULATE THE BODY

Ambergris, cinnamon bun and other food aromas, jasmine, musks, neroli, patchouli, rose, sandalwood, and ylang-ylang are natural erotic scents that have a physical (usually hormonal) effect that may enhance sex. Most of these have additional emotional benefits, as well.

### *Ambergris*

*Aroma:* Sweet, mild, pleasant, earthy

Readers of *Moby Dick* will be familiar with ambergris, the highly prized, sweetly scented product of a sperm whale. It is sometimes found floating on tropical seas or washed up in lumps (ranging from .05 oz to 200 lb) on the shore. In Asia, ambergris is used as an aphrodisiac. It is called *lung sien hiang*, "dragon's spittle perfume," because it was once thought to be the drool of dragons who slept on rocks by the sea. Actually, it is the vomit of the sperm whale, caused by intestinal irritation from the beaks of squid it has eaten.

Whale vomit does not seem a likely substance to conjure up romantic feelings, but strangely enough, it has a wonderful fragrance. Ambergris is very rare and expensive. It is used in fine perfumes to prolong and soften floral fragrances. The scent of ambergris is so tenacious that it will remain on the skin for several days, in spite of repeated washings. A single drop placed in a book still remained fragrant after forty years. It is also reputed to be a powerful aphrodisiac when taken by mouth. In Asia, ambergris-laced coffee is still used for this purpose.

The famous eighteenth-century writer James Boswell claimed that a mere 3 grains (0.194 grams) would arouse lust in a camel. Just one gram, and an elephant would be mad with desire.

Like other animal-based scents, ambergris is available only in synthetic form. It is sold as a fragrant oil by manufacturers of aromatherapy products and is also an ingredient in many floral perfumes.

### Cinnamon Bun *(and other food aromas)*

*Aroma:* Warm, pleasant, sweet, spicy

The way to a man's heart is through his stomach—via food aromas, according to Dr. Alan R. Hirsch, a neurologist at the Smell and Taste Treatment and Research Foundation of Chicago. According to his research, aromas such as the smell of cinnamon buns are sexually stimulating and may be useful aphrodisiacs.

Hirsch says, "Perfumes have been used for centuries to elicit sexual arousal, yet no scientific study has ever been conducted to prove their effectiveness. We set out to explore the effects of odors on penile blood flow with the hope that positive results would aid in the treatment of impotence."

To test which scents arouse men most, Dr. Hirsch measured the effects of different odors on blood flow to the penis. The test was conducted with thirty-one volunteers, who tested forty-six scents and a variety of combinations by sniffing through scented masks. Neither the "smellers" nor the test administrators knew which scents were being tested. Scents included a variety of fragrances (e.g., musk, rose, lily of the valley, lavender, and baby powder) as well as numerous food aromas (e.g., freshly baked cinnamon buns, pumpkin pie, pizza, roasting meat, and buttered popcorn).

The results? None of the odors *decreased* blood flow to the penis. All odors had some positive effect, but some odors were much more arousing than others. Least arousing was the odor of cranberries, which only increased blood flow 2 percent. The aromas of baby powder, parsley, and roses were only slightly more stimulating.

Scoring higher on the sensual scale were pizza, doughnuts, and oranges. The top three winners were combination odors: (1) pumpkin pie and lavender; (2) doughnuts and licorice; (3) pumpkin pie and licorice. All three *significantly* increased penile blood flow.

The top winner, pumpkin pie and lavender, increased penile blood flow an average of 40 percent.

The study also found that:

- *Lavender* was the most sexually stimulating scent for men whose sexual partners usually wore a fragrance.
- Those who felt satisfied sexually were most aroused by the scent of *strawberries*.
- *Vanilla* was the most sexually stimulating scent for older men.
- The most sexually active men in the group found the odors of *lavender*, *cola*, and *oriental spice* the most sexually stimulating.

Overall, the results were impressive enough to suggest that scents may be useful as aphrodisiacs and also as a treatment for vasculogenic impotence, which is related to penile blood flow.

A cinnamon-bun fragrance is already commercially available, made by Frontier Herbs of Norway, Iowa. Lavender, vanilla, and strawberry are readily obtainable since they are basic oils and fragrances in aromatherapy.

## Jasmine (*Jasminum officinale* or *J. grandiflorum*)

*Aroma:* Exotic, intoxicating, full, rich, heavy, sweet

Since ancient times the intoxicating scent of jasmine has been praised for its aphrodisiac powers by both men and women. Jasmine has a heavy, sensual, almost animal quality that is similar to musk in its aphrodisiac effects. Known as the king of fragrances, jasmine is far more powerful and masculine than its queen, the rose. It is a component of virtually every fine fragrance, floral or masculine—and its effects as an aphrodisiac are both physical and emotional.

Jasmine is one of the finest fragrances available, but it is expensive. It takes eight million blossoms to produce a kilogram of oil, and the blossoms can only be gathered at night, when the fragrance is at its peak. Extraction of the oil is labor-intensive and involves layering the blossoms on panes of fat-covered glass and then melting the fat to extract the aromatic compounds. Because of jasmine's exorbitant price, most commercial fragrances use synthetic jasmine, which has an overly sweet quality. True jasmine is available as an essential oil for aromatherapy. In aromatherapy it is used as a fragrance to be inhaled, or it is mixed with a massage oil.

Jasmine is said to strengthen the male sexual organs. In aromatherapy, it is used to treat impotence, low libido, and prostate problems.

As an emotional booster, jasmine is superb. It is a stimulant and antidepressant, valuable for promoting an emotional climate conducive to sex. Jasmine's reputation is supported by research. It was tested and proven effective as an antidepressant by Italian researcher Paolo Rovesti. Aromatherapists say that jasmine represents passion and joy. Its aroma engenders a feeling of well-being, boosts confidence and optimism, and reduces lethargy caused by depression.

The aroma of jasmine is a mental stimulant as well. Professor Shizuo Torii and colleagues at Toho University in Tokyo found that jasmine increases alertness and attention by stimulating certain types of brain-wave activity.

Frontier Cooperative Herbs, which sells true jasmine oil, suggests that an inexpensive and natural way to enjoy the fragrance of jasmine is to grow the living plant. It requires rich, moist, well-drained soil, but is relatively easy to grow. A single plant will strongly scent an entire room or patio on a still summer's eve.

Other uses: Jasmine oil, mixed with a massage oil, is applied as a treatment for dry or sensitive skin, wrinkles, and to rejuvenate aging skin. It is also diluted and rubbed on temples to relieve headaches.

### The Musks

*Aroma:* Musky, dark, masculine, animal-like

Musk has been called the fragrance of sex, the universal aphrodisiac. Its name is derived from the Sanskrit word for testicle, and in nature it is a type of scent produced by males. Actually, musk is not a single scent, but rather a general term for musky-type odors produced by the breaking down of male hormones. Curiously, musk is an aphrodisiac for both males and females. Musk is also used in the plant world to attract pollinators, as for example, by musk melons, musk hyacinths, musk orchids, musk pears, musk seeds, muscatels, and the musk rose.

Musk was originally obtained from an abdominal gland of the male musk deer. Today its synthetic forms are usually used, galaxolide and Exaltolide. Natural musk oil contains the male pheromone alpha-androstenol, so it arouses through the VNO as well as through the sense of smell. Some perfume manufacturers capitalize on this connection, producing products that contain alpha-androstenol. An intriguing discussion of musk and other hormone-related sex attractants can be found in *The Scent of Eros* by Kohl and Francoeur, a valuable resource for anyone interested in the connection between sex and the sense of smell.

## Neroli *(Citrus aurantium, C. vulgaris)*

*Aroma:* Fresh, floral, spicy, refreshing, sweet

Neroli is the fragrance of orange blossoms. It was named for the seventeenth-century Italian princess of Neroli, Anna Maria de la Tremoille, who introduced the fragrance to her native France. The sensual aroma of orange blossoms has been used as an aphrodisiac since ancient times. It was one of the fragrances loved and used by Cleopatra.

Neroli's exquisite fragrance is relaxing, soothing, and at the same time uplifting to the spirit. It reduces anxiety connected with sex and induces self-confidence and a mild euphoria. These qualities make it a perfect fragrance to set the stage for love. It is no accident that orange blossoms are included in the traditional bridal bouquet. In times past, orange blossoms and rose petals were scattered throughout the bridal chamber to disperse their sensuous scents to the lovers.

Neroli is expensive, as it takes a ton of orange blossoms to produce a quart of neroli oil. A less expensive alternative is pettigrain, a fragrance very similar to neroli, which is produced by distilling the leaves of the orange tree rather than its blossoms.

Other uses: Neroli is used as an inhalant or as a bath oil to induce sleep, for relaxation, and to treat grief or depression. It is mixed with a base oil, such as grapeseed or sweet almond, and massaged into the skin to improve elasticity, treat scars, prevent stretch marks, and improve circulation.

## Patchouli *(Pogostemon patchouli)*

*Aroma:* Animal-like, musky, pungent, penetrating, persistent

Patchouli has been used as an aphrodisiac for centuries. It was a favorite ingredient for love potions and charms and was reputed to have magical powers. The sensual aroma of patchouli supposedly releases inhibitions and encourages lovers to communicate their sexual needs. According to aromatherapists, patchouli affects the pituitary gland, which, among other things, stimulates hormone production. Patchouli's aphrodisiac properties only work, of course, if both partners like it.

Patchouli's fragrance improves with age, like fine wine. It loses its sour quality and becomes more balsamic. Its aroma is persistent and can remain in clothing even after several washings.

Other uses: In aromatherapy, patchouli is used as an inhalant for its calming and antidepressant qualities and to "sharpen the wits." Some say it helps combat obesity. In Asia, it is used to repel moths. Mixed with a base oil, patchouli is applied externally to treat dry, wrinkled skin and such problems as seborrhea, acne, and dermatitis.

## Rose *(Rosa damascena, R. centifolia)*

*Aroma:* Sweet, floral, warm, intense, rich, evocative

Throughout the ages rose has been a precious fragrance, the perfume of pharaohs and kings. Known as the queen of fragrances, rose has been used since ancient times in religious and magical ceremonies and as an aphrodisiac—especially for women. It was a favorite ingredient in love potions. Ancient herbalists classified the rose as an herb of Venus, the planet that rules the sexual organs and sexual love. In ancient Rome, roses were strewn in the path of the bridal party at weddings, and rose petals were scattered on the bridal bed.

The fragrance of rose has always been the fragrance of love, designed to entice and seduce a lover. Legend has it that when Cleopatra met Antony, she had her bedroom carpeted with fresh rose petals an inch deep. But the prize for most extravagant use of roses for sensual pleasure undoubtedly goes to the Roman emperor Nero. His escapade with roses is described by Kathi Keville and Mindy Green in their *Aromatherapy: A Complete Guide to the Healing Art.*

The authors tell how Nero spent the equivalent of $100,000 to install concealed pipes in the carved ivory ceilings of his dining rooms for a single party he held in A.D. 54. Fragrant mists were sprayed from the pipes to the guests below, and sliding panels opened to shower them with rose petals. Unfortunately, Nero went overboard on the rose petals, and one guest reportedly suffocated in them, dying a bizarre— but fragrant—death.

Today, rose continues to be one of the most highly valued and expensive fragrances. The process of extracting the essential fragrance from the flowers is extremely costly. A ton of rose petals yields about a pound of essential rose oil. Yet despite its cost, rose fragrance is in high demand. It is a component in 48 percent of men's fragrances and 98 percent of women's. In every type of perfume, rose lends beauty and depth to the aroma.

Rose works as an aphrodisiac for several reasons. First is the sensual appeal of the fragrance itself. Second are its evocative properties. Rose is such a popular fragrance and flower that one is bound to have memories associated with it—and those memories may well be erotic. Finally, rose is an emotional aphrodisiac that promotes feelings of well-being and happiness—possibly because it contains phenyl ethanol, which has narcotic properties. It reduces anxiety connected with sex and may be helpful in treating impotence or difficulty in becoming aroused for emotional reasons.

Other uses: The scent of rose is inhaled to treat headaches, depression, emotional shock, or grief. Rose oil, mixed with a base oil, is applied topically to treat conditions such as eczema, wrinkles, dryness, and congested pores.

In *The Art of Sensual Aromatherapy*, Nitya Lacroix advises that the essential oil of rose is best avoided during pregnancy.

## Sandalwood *(Santalum album)*

*Aroma:* Musky, deep, woody, masculine, sweet, tenacious

Sandalwood is a musky fragrance that smells very much like alpha-androstenol, a male pheromone present in human sweat. This may help explain why sandalwood has been considered an aphrodisiac since ancient times. In addition, sandalwood is a hormone regulator and affects the pituitary gland.

Sandalwood is one of the few fragrances that is equally popular among both men and women. As an aphrodisiac its fragrance works on the emotions as well as the body. It is an antidepressant and creates mild euphoria and a sense of well-being. In aromatherapy it is often used to treat impotence.

## Ylang-Ylang *(Cananga odorata)*

*Aroma:* Extremely sweet, soft, floral, sensual

Ylang-ylang's reputation as an aphrodisiac is due primarily to its effect on the emotions, although its aroma does stimulate the adrenal glands. The fragrance of ylang-ylang acts as an antidepressant. It soothes stress and anxiety—two prime sources of sexual difficulties—and calms the emotions.

Ylang-ylang means "flower of flowers," a fitting name because the flowers of this tree have an extremely sweet, heavy, sensual aroma. Some people find the aroma too heavy and sweet. Thus ylang-ylang is sometimes mixed with other oils, such as bergamot or lemon. Ylang-ylang is often used in massage oils as well as in perfumes, colognes, and incense.

Other uses: Ylang-ylang fragrance is inhaled to treat insomnia, to reduce blood pressure, and to slow rapid breathing or rapid heart rate.

Using too high a concentration of ylang-ylang or using it for too long can cause nausea and/or headache.

# SCENTS TO ENHANCE
# MOOD AND THE EMOTIONS

❧

When you want to have sex but you are too tired or anxious, a fragrance may help to put you in the mood. These charts list fragrances and oils that are readily available. Most are sold as essential oils, which are used in aromatherapy.

## SCENTS THAT STIMULATE

| | |
|---|---|
| Basil<br>(*Ocimum*<br>*basilicum*) | EFFECTS Stimulating, awakens the senses, arousing, relieves fatigue.<br>AROMA Spicy, slight camphor tone.<br>CAUTIONS Avoid during pregnancy. Avoid if you have sensitive skin. |
| Bergamot<br>(*Citrus*<br>*bergamia*) | EFFECTS Uplifting, an antidepressant, refreshing.<br>AROMA Lemony, floral, spicy.<br>CAUTIONS Increases skin's photosensitivity. Do not use before going out in the sun. Use Bergamot FCF, which doesn't have this effect. |
| Coriander<br>(*Coriandrum*<br>*sativum*) | EFFECTS Warming, stimulating, a druid "lust potion."<br>AROMA Warm, woodsy, spicy, fruity.<br>CAUTIONS Use in moderation. |
| Frankincense<br>(*Boswellia*<br>*carteri*) | EFFECTS Heightens awareness, aids communication, stimulates the senses.<br>AROMA Warm, resinous, similar to balsam. |
| Lemon<br>(*Citrus*<br>*limonum*) | EFFECTS Fortifies the nervous system.<br>AROMA Clear, citrusy, sharp, refreshing. |
| Pepper<br>(*Piper nigrum*) | EFFECTS Warming, stimulating, arouses the senses.<br>AROMA Sharp, spicy. |
| Vanilla<br>(*Vanilla*<br>*planifolia*) | EFFECTS Warming, stimulating, arousing, evocative.<br>AROMA Rich, sweet, liked by both men and women. |

## SCENTS THAT SOOTHE

Ambretta
(*Hibiscus abel-moschus*)

EFFECTS Relieves anxiety, depression, nervous tension.
AROMA Strong, floral-musky, lingering.

Cedarwood
(*Cedrus atlantica*)

EFFECTS Soothing, evocative, relieves fears and tensions.
AROMA Dry, masculine, woody.
CAUTIONS Avoid during pregnancy.

Chamomile
(*Anthemis nobilis*)

EFFECTS Calming, soothing, relieves depression, relaxing.
AROMA Refreshing, slightly bitter.
CAUTIONS Can cause dermatitis.

Clary Sage
(*Salvia sclarea*)

EFFECTS Relaxing, euphoric, decreases inhibitions, mildly intoxicating.
AROMA Sweet, dry, strong, nutty.
CAUTIONS Avoid during pregnancy. Do not use with alcohol.

Lavender
(*Lavandula angustifolia*)

EFFECTS Very relaxing, relieves nervous tension.
AROMA Refreshing, woody tones.
CAUTIONS Avoid in first trimester of pregnancy.

# CHAPTER SIX

## *Food as Aphrodisiacs*

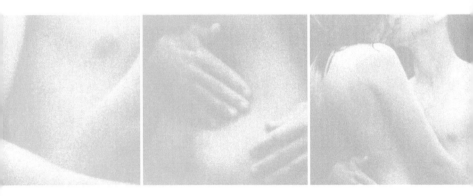

*Y*ou share a very intimate relationship with your food. As the saying goes, "You are what you eat." (Or as Dom DeLuise once put it, "Look at me. I'm a Twinkie!") Since there is such a powerful cause-and-effect relationship between what you eat and what you will become, it follows that you need to pay attention to your diet. For peak performance, you need high-grade nutrients. This is as true for sex as it is for any high-energy activity. For an active, satisfying sex life you need optimum health and optimum nutrition.

Food affects sexuality both directly and indirectly. Certain nutrients boost levels of hormones and neurotransmitters that create sexual arousal and increase the flow of blood to the sexual organs. Others affect sex indirectly by influencing levels of hormones and neurotransmitters that have a powerful effect on the emotions. Nutrients can trigger the release of hormones and neurotransmitters that promote—or thwart—the desire to make love.

As with herbs and essential oils, some nutrients have gained a "sexy" reputation. These are taken prior to lovemaking for a temporary, short-term burst of sexual desire and energy. Other nutrients work for the long term to increase overall sexual vigor and vitality, by fortifying glands and the reproductive organs and by affecting levels of sex hormones and neurotransmitters.

## ❧ NUTRIENTS TAKEN PRIOR TO LOVEMAKING

Ordinarily, nutrients take some time to do their job. Their effects on the body may not be noticeable for weeks or even months. This holds true for most nutrients that enhance sex. Some, however, are fast acting and are taken a short time prior to lovemaking for their stimulating effect. These sex-enhancing nutrients are available in certain foods and also as nutritional supplements.

Following is a list of fast-acting nutrients.

### Vitamin E (Tocopherol)

Topping the list is vitamin E, the most-hyped vitamin of the decade. Popularly referred to as the "sex vitamin" or "virility vitamin," this vitamin's popularity as a sex booster led one wit to recommend that it be reclassified as a "recreational drug."

Vitamin E's many advocates say that it is a source of high energy, an almost-instant rejuvenator. They claim that taking a high-potency vitamin-E capsule a half-hour before sex results in a flood of sexual energy that lasts for several hours. Vitamin E supplies not only energy, but endurance.

Like most other reputed sex-boosters, vitamin E has not had its aphrodisiac properties studied. Evidence that it works as an aphrodisiac is anecdotal. However, these claims may be valid.

Vitamin E is a powerful antioxidant. This means that it prevents substances in the body from oxidizing and being converted to free radicals, toxic molecules that do extensive damage to cells. By thus protecting red blood cells from free radicals, Vitamin E enables them to carry their full supply of pure oxygen throughout the body.

Every cell in the body needs oxygen for optimum performance. When our cells are deficient in oxygen we become fatigued. We lack endurance. It follows that we have little energy for sex, or any other activity requiring an increased expenditure of oxygen.

Vitamin E is also vital to energy metabolism. Working with coenzyme Q10, it helps convert the food we eat into energy.

Vitamin E is called the virility vitamin for good reason. It is essential to the production of sperm, sex hormones, and gonadotropin—a pituitary hormone that stimulates the sex glands. In male laboratory animals, an inadequate supply of vitamin E resulted in a decreased level of sex hormones and in the degeneration of testicles.

Test tube studies have shown that vitamin E increases the fertility and motility (spontaneous motion) of human sperm. The potency and activity of sperm are in direct proportion to the amount of vitamin E in a man's semen.

Food sources: Wheat germ, cold-pressed vegetable oils, whole grains, leafy green vegetables, nuts, seeds, liver, eggs.

If you have high blood pressure, do not take vitamin E without first consulting your physician. Large doses of vitamin E may increase blood pressure.

## L-Arginine

L-arginine is one of eight essential amino acids. The term "essential" is slightly misleading because it suggests that some amino acids are nonessential to the body, which is not true. Essential amino acids are those that the body cannot synthesize on its own, and therefore must be included in the diet.

L-arginine works as a sex-booster by increasing the neuro-transmitters that cause sexual arousal. It also plays a crucial role in the satisfaction one obtains from sex.

L-arginine is a favorite of body builders and athletes, who use it for increasing muscle mass and reducing fat. L-arginine causes the release of growth hormone from the pituitary glands. Growth hormone stimulates muscle growth and at the same time boosts metabolism in the fat cells, causing them to burn up more body fat. Athletes say that L-arginine also gives them more energy, stamina, and endurance.

Recently L-arginine has been found to play a major role in a man's ability to have an erection. When a man is sexually stimulated, it sets up a chain reaction in which an enzyme converts L-arginine in the penis to nitric oxide. Nitric oxide, in turn, triggers an erection. The ability to have an erection is directly related to the amount of L-arginine and oxygen carried by the blood to the penis.

L-arginine occurs naturally in many foods. It is also taken as a nutritional supplement by both men and women. Although L-arginine supplementation is generally safe, one aggravating side effect can occur. If a herpes virus is present in the body, an increase in L-arginine can reactivate it. This can be countered by taking equal amounts of lysine and L-arginine. Lysine is an amino acid that reduces the growth of viruses, such as the herpes virus that causes cold sores and the herpes virus that causes genital herpes. The high L-arginine content in peanuts and in chocolate explains why some people get cold sores after bingeing on them. Anyone prone to outbreaks of cold sores or genital herpes would do well to take lysine supplements.

Food sources: Brown rice, peanuts, nuts, chocolate, poultry, raisins, dairy products, sesame seeds, sunflower seeds, oatmeal, popcorn, carob, raw cereal, whole-wheat products.

Because L-arginine releases growth hormone, it should not be used by young people whose bones are still growing.

Supplemental L-arginine should not be taken by anyone with kidney or liver disease.

L-arginine and other amino-acid supplements should not be taken by women who are pregnant or lactating.

### Choline and Lecithin (Phosphatidylcholine)

Choline is usually classified as one of the B vitamins. It is crucial in the transmission of chemical messages between the nerves and brain, including those that elevate mood. Choline is essential for sexual arousal and may also boost sexual performance.

Choline is the main component of lecithin, a fatty acid that protects cell membranes from hardening and being damaged by oxygen. Semen contains large amounts of lecithin, which must be replaced after ejaculation.

Choline stimulates the brain to produce and release the neurotransmitter acetylcholine. Acetylcholine elevates mood and stimulates sexual arousal, especially for those over the age of forty, when choline levels in the cells may begin to decline. Acetylcholine also triggers the release of lubricating moisture from the mucous membranes of the vagina in preparation for sexual intercourse. It helps men maintain an erection and aids in hormone production.

When used to arouse desire, 100 to 200 mg of choline is taken a half hour before having sex.

Choline also boosts brain power—especially memory—and aids weight-loss by emulsifying fats so they can be flushed from the cells.

Some people prefer taking lecithin supplements rather than choline because they say that choline gives them a "fishy" body odor. Lecithin granules provide a convenient way to take choline as a daily supplement. The granules dissolve easily in juice, tea, or soup, or they can be sprinkled over food or added to a bread mix. Some users say that lecithin makes tea more satisfying. This is probably because of its oil content. Two tablespoons a day of the granules should be sufficient.

Food sources: Egg yolks, liver, soybeans, fish, meat, milk, whole-grain cereals, peas, beans, peanuts, seeds, nuts, green vegetables, brewer's yeast.

Megadoses of choline may aggravate depression.

Choline may cause diarrhea.

Do not take choline supplements if you have gastric ulcers or Parkinson's disease, or if you are taking prescription drugs such as atropine or diphenhydramine, which are meant to block the effects of acetylcholine.

### Phenylalanine and Tyrosine

We have seen how choline enhances sex by increasing production of the sex-boosting neurotransmitter acetylcholine. The amino acids phenylalanine and tyrosine increase levels of two other sex-boosting brain neurotransmitters, norepinephrine and dopamine.

Phenylalanine is an essential amino acid that exists in two forms: D-phenylalanine (taken for pain) and L-phenylalanine

## HOW TO TAKE AMINO ACID SUPPLEMENTS

✿

When taking an individual amino acid supplement such as tyrosine, take it on an empty stomach to aid absorption, since the different amino acids compete with each other to enter the brain. Tyrosine, for example, competes with tryptophan, an amino acid used by the body to make serotonin. Tyrosine is an "upper"; tryptophan is a "downer." If tyrosine enters the brain first, it primes the brain for alertness, stimulates memory and mental function, and promotes an elevated mood. If tryptophan enters the brain first, it can slow down reaction time, cause sleepiness or lethargy, and even induce depression.

(taken for depression). The nutritional supplement DLPA (DL-phenylalanine) combines both types. According to Durk Pearson and Sandy Shaw, authors of *Life Extension*, DLPA is the best form to take. They also note that in clinical tests, phenylalanine was twice as effective for depression as the prescription drug imipramine.

Tyrosine, like L-phenylalanine, is an antidepressant. When low sex drive is related to depression, nutrients that attack depression can help. Tyrosine also increases levels of neurotransmitters that control sex drive. Tyrosine is a nonessential amino acid because it can be manufactured by the body from phenylalanine. Both tyrosine and phenylalanine are available as nonprescription supplements.

Food sources: Lean red meat, poultry, seafood, soybeans, wheat germ, dairy products, nuts, seeds.

Phenylalanine and tyrosine are stimulating to some people and may cause insomnia and anxiety. Avoid taking them if you are taking antidepressants or an MAO inhibitor or if you have high blood pressure, phenylketonuria, melanoma skin cancer, or diabetes.

### Phenylethylamine (PEA)

Phenylethylamine, or PEA, is the chemical of romance, the chemical that ignites "love at first sight." It is called the "molecule of love." PEA is made in the brain from phenylalanine. Its production is triggered by thoughts of sex or romance.

PEA is a natural amphetamine, a mood elevator for both sexes. It produces excitement, euphoria, the thrill of romance. Sometimes its effects appear to be instant, to happen in a flash. When you are "struck by cupid's arrow" the tip of that arrow is most likely impregnated with PEA. It is the release of PEA that creates "love at first sight," the feeling of being "smitten." Under the spell of PEA, the delicious feelings intensify; they peak at orgasm and return at the thought or sight of the beloved. When you are high on PEA there is an underlying excitement to life, a sense of anticipation.

Like other amphetamine highs, a PEA high can be habit forming. People can become addicted to the feelings associated with falling in love. ("Falling in love with love," as the song goes.) If their romance falls apart these people don't simply get the blues, they develop acute physical symptoms similar to amphetamine withdrawal. They are miserable emotionally and physically. They need their PEA fix. If a romantic replacement is not in the immediate picture, they often "gorge" on chocolate—not for its sugar content or its taste or its small amount of caffeine, but for its PEA content.

A craving for chocolate can be a hunger for love and the emotional highs associated with it. The PEA in chocolate helps to recreate these feelings to some degree. After the breakup of a love affair, people often take refuge in chocolate.

Are there other, less-fattening food sources of PEA? No. However, there is the artificial food sweetener Nutrasweet, which the body can convert to PEA. Nutrasweet is found in many brands of diet soda, diet chewing gum, and other diet foods.

PEA levels can also be increased by sexual or romantic fantasies, reading romance novels, listening to romantic music, or reliving a romantic memory. Erotic novels, X-rated films, erotic art, and other sexually explicit material can also raise PEA levels.

## ～ NUTRIENTS TAKEN REGULARLY FOR LONG-TERM SEXUAL VIGOR

The arousal-enhancing nutrients described above also enhance long-term sexual vigor. There are others. Of special importance are certain essential fatty acids, the entire vitamin B-complex, and certain minerals. In addition, there is the matter of calories. Calories in food provide energy for all our activities—including sex.

### *Getting the Right Amount of Calories*

Anorexia is not sexy. Like any other worthwhile physical activity, sex requires calories—lots of them. Thin may be in, but going on a starvation diet to make yourself sexually irresistible can easily backfire. When you eat too few calories, your sex drive disappears along with your unwanted pounds. Even if you reach your ideal physical goal you may be too tired or irritable to make love. This is not to discourage you from losing weight, but to caution you against trying to lose it "instantly" with an extremely low-calorie fad diet that is a nutritional disaster.

The "starve and be sexy" approach is self-defeating. What about the opposite approach: "The more there is of me, the more there is to love!" Is that view simply a self-deceiving rationalization? Perhaps not. As Anita Ekberg commented, "I'm very much bigger than I was, so what? It's not really fatness, it's development" (*Daily Mail*, September 2, 1972).

Being overweight does not necessarily lower a person's sex appeal. But while excess weight may not stand in the way of romance, it can adversely affect the body's reproductive system. It even affects production of sex hormones. This is particularly true when overweight is the result of a high-fat diet.

Fat produces estrogen, the primary female hormone. For women, this inadvertent accumulation of excess estrogen can cause unpleasant side effects such as disturbed menstrual cycles and bloating. It can also increase the risk of developing breast cancer, since that cancer is estrogen-dependent. This risk can be reduced by avoiding high-fat foods.

For men, a diet that is high in fat leads to a body that is low in testosterone, the hormone responsible for sex drive. A study at the University of Utah tested the effect of high fat on the testosterone levels of eight male volunteers. The results were astonishing. After drinking high-fat milkshakes (57 percent fat, 34 percent carbohydrates, 9 percent protein) the men's testosterone levels dropped approximately 50 percent. When they drank low-fat milkshakes (1 percent fat, 73 percent carbohydrates, 25 percent protein) their testosterone levels did not decline at all. The researchers concluded that over a period of time a high-fat diet can deplete a man's sex drive. Their conclusion has been supported by other studies.

In addition to lowering libido, a high-fat diet may contribute to atherosclerosis, the build-up of fatty plaque deposits in the blood vessels, including the numerous tiny blood vessels in the penis. When the blood vessels are narrowed by plaque deposits, they cannot supply the penis with the amount of blood needed to achieve an erection; nor can they respond to sexual signals governed by the sex drive.

A diet that is high in animal fats—especially fat found in red meat—may affect hormone levels of both men and women. Female hormones are frequently added to the food of grazing animals such as beef cattle and also sometimes to chickens to fatten them up more quickly for market. As women are well aware, female hormones cause the body to retain water and put on weight. Although the public has been assured that any resulting amounts of female hormones in the meat are insignificant, not everyone is comfortable with this assurance. American beef has been banned in some countries because of this practice.

This is not to say that you must eliminate all fat for the health of your hormones. To do so would be disastrous to your skin. It would also prevent fat-soluble vitamins from being used by the body: vitamins A, D, E, and K. You need to have some fat in your diet, but the healthiest sources are vegetables, nuts, seeds, and fish oil. Included in these necessary fats are the essential fatty acids.

### Essential Fatty Acids

Essential fatty acids are fats the body needs but cannot manufacture on its own. It is essential that they be supplied in the diet. Essential fatty acids serve many important functions that include:

- Strengthening cell membranes
- Promoting growth of muscles and nerves
- Reducing levels of cholesterol and blood fat

They are also crucial to your sex life. Essential fatty acids are needed for:

- The normal functioning of your sex organs and glands
- The production of sex hormones and adrenal hormones
- Stimulating the production of *prostaglandins*—hormone-like substances vital to sexual response (sometimes injected locally to treat impotence)
- Improving circulation, which enables blood to flow into the genitals and aids erections

The two essential fatty acids that perform these functions are linoleic acid and EPA (eicosapentaenoic acid). The best sources of linoleic acid are cold-pressed oils of vegetables, seeds, and nuts. EPA is part of the omega-3 group of fatty acids, which are found in the oil of fish, such as salmon, that live in deep, cold, fresh water. The omega-3 fish oils are extremely effective in lowering cholesterol and blood fat levels, thereby improving circulation and thinning the blood.

Both linoleic acid and EPA produce prostaglandins, which are critical to sexual response and to male erections. In order to produce prostaglandins, however, these fatty acids must have an adequate supply of vitamins $B_3$ and $B_6$, vitamin C, zinc, and magnesium.

Food sources: *Linoleic acid:* Safflower oil, sunflower oil, evening primrose oil, black currant oil, soy oil, corn oil, sesame oil, walnuts, almonds, peanut butter.

*EPA omega-3:* Salmon, mackerel, menhaden, herring, sardines, flaxseed oil.

EPA should not be used if you are taking blood-thinning medication. When excessive amounts of EPA are taken, it can reduce the ability of the blood to form clots.

In *Prescription for Nutritional Healing*, James F. Balch and Phyllis A. Balch advise diabetics to eat fish for its essentially fatty acids, but to avoid taking fish-oil supplements.

### Vitamin B-Complex

Fast food, processed food, junk food—all seem to be an integral and perhaps necessary part of today's fast-paced lifestyle. Yet convenience and instant satisfaction have their price in less than optimal health and vitamin deficiencies. Among the most common of these are deficiencies of the B vitamins, deficiencies that were quick to emerge following that highly touted, highly processed innovation—white bread. Until that time, whole grains had been the main source of B vitamins in the average diet. But most of the B vitamins are removed in the process of making white bread. Without the basic B vitamins, bread is no longer the "staff of life." There are, of course, other factors that cause deficiencies of the B vitamins, such as age and certain health problems.

If you are deficient in any of the B vitamins it is almost impossible to have a fulfilling sex life. The reason can be summed up in two words: energy and nerves. Without the B vitamins your body could not convert carbohydrates into glucose—a simple sugar that is the body's chief source of energy. Nor could you metabolize (break down) fats or proteins. In short, even though you ate, you would get no energy from your food.

Vitamin B deficiency can also result in irritability, even to the point of aggressiveness and nervousness, the feeling of being "on edge."

Unless you eat a lot of wheat germ, whole grains, brewer's yeast, or liver, it is almost impossible to obtain sufficient B vitamins from food alone. On the other hand, if you take supplements of a single B vitamin, the need for the other B vitamins is greatly increased. A surplus of one of the B vitamins could cause a deficiency of another. Thus it is a good policy to take a balanced vitamin B-complex supplement.

The following section describes the B vitamins that are most important to your love life. Be sure your diet is adequately supplied with these energy-giving, mood-elevating nutrients.

# IMPORTANT B VITAMINS

## VITAMIN

**Vitamin $B_1$**
(*Thiamine*)

EFFECTS  The "morale" vitamin. Converts carbohydrates to energy. Combats fatigue and depression. A deficiency of this vitamin drains your energy and sex life.
SOURCES  Wheat germ, brewer's yeast, bran, legumes, nuts and seeds, liver, kidney, pork, fish

**Vitamin $B_2$**
(*Riboflavin*)

EFFECTS  Vital to energy. Helps metabolize carbohydrates and proteins. Essential for production of hormones by the adrenal glands.
SOURCES  Liver, dairy products, beans, eggs, fish, poultry, spinach, wheat germ, brewer's yeast

**Vitamin $B_3$**
(*Niacin*)

EFFECTS  Vital to energy. Helps metabolize carbohydrates and fats. Combats fatigue, depression, anxiety, insomnia. Enhances sex by dilating blood vessels to promote blood flow to the brain and to the sexual organs.
SOURCES  Chicken, liver, salmon, kidney, peanuts, brewer's yeast, chickpeas, brown rice, seeds
CAUTION  May cause flushed skin. (Avoid by using "no-flush" niacin.) Overdoses may cause: liver damage, higher levels of uric acid, higher levels of blood sugar.

**Vitamin $B_5$**
(*Pantothenic acid*)

EFFECTS  The anti-stress vitamin. Helps metabolize carbohydrates and fat. Combats fatigue, depression, and anxiety.
SOURCES  Beans, beef, eggs, pork, fish, vegetables, whole wheat
CAUTION  Extremely high doses may cause diarrhea or water retention.

Vitamin B$_6$
(*Pyridoxine*)

EFFECTS  Used in the synthesis of the neuro-transmitter epinephrine, which is involved in orgasm. Combats depression, mood swings, PMS (premenstrual syndrome), water retention. Helps metabolize fats, proteins, and carbohydrates.
SOURCES  Brewer's yeast, chicken, liver, pork, fish, whole grains, sunflower seeds, wheat germ, potatoes, dried beans, bananas
CAUTION  Excessive intake may cause deterioration of sensory nerves (nerves that transmit information for sight, hearing, etc.).

Vitamin B$_{12}$
(*Cyanocobalamin*)

EFFECTS  Helps metabolize carbohydrates and fats. Essential for production of red blood cells. Prevents nerve damage. A deficiency of this vitamin decreases the sex drive.
SOURCES  Liver, chicken, beef, pork, fish, clams, eggs, dairy products (found only in animal products)

Folic Acid

EFFECTS  Vital for energy and formation of red blood cells. Helps metabolize proteins. Combats fatigue, irritability, depression.
SOURCES  Green leafy vegetables, broccoli, liver, mushrooms, nuts, beans, bran, brewer's yeast
CAUTION  Large doses may inhibit absorption of zinc. Epileptics taking phenytoin should not take folic acid, which inhibits absorption of that drug.

## Minerals

Starting as minute particles of rocks and stone that form the basis of soil, minerals are passed:

- From soil to plants
- From plants to plant-eating animals
- From plants and plant-eating animals to us—eaters of both plants and animals

Of all the nutrients, minerals are the most vital to our survival. The body can function without vitamins, but not without minerals. Even vitamins need the presence of minerals in order to do their work. Minerals are required by all the body's cells and for the functioning of body processes such as digestion and, of course, sex. Without minerals even bodily fluids, including semen, cannot be produced. Minerals are chemical catalysts that make things happen.

There are two groups of minerals. First are the *macro-* (bulk) minerals that we need in larger quantities: calcium, magnesium, sodium, potassium, phosphorous. Second are the *micro-* (trace) minerals that we need in minute quantities: zinc, iron, copper, manganese, chromium, selenium, iodine.

Excess minerals are stored in bones and muscles, so it is possible to overdose on them if you take large quantities over a long period of time.

Minerals compete for absorption in the body. A high dosage of zinc, for example, can deplete calcium or copper. Thus it is best not to take single mineral supplements except under the guidance of a health professional.

Mineral supplements are available in chelated form. This means they are attached to a protein to aid absorption. When you take a mineral supplement with a meal, however, the minerals are usually chelated automatically in the stomach during digestion. (Do not take a fiber supplement with the same meal because the extra fiber will interfere with mineral absorption.)

The following chart describes the effects of certain minerals on our sex lives.

# IMPORTANT MINERALS

❧

<u>MINERAL</u>

Calcium      <u>EFFECTS</u> Combats nervous tension and irritability.
<u>SOURCES</u> Dairy products, sardines, seaweed, green leafy vegetables, almonds, molasses.
<u>CAUTION</u> Excessive intake of calcium may interfere with iron absorption. It may cause abdominal pain or calcium deposits in tissues.

Chromium      <u>EFFECTS</u> Vital to energy. Aids in metabolizing glucose for energy and in regulating blood sugar levels.
<u>SOURCES</u> Brewer's yeast, liver, beef, potatoes, cheese, whole grains

Iodine      <u>EFFECTS</u> Vital to energy. Essential to the thyroid gland which regulates basal metabolism, the speed at which body activities occur. A deficiency can weaken the sex drive and create fatigue.
<u>SOURCES</u> Iodized salt, seafood, kelp, onions, pineapple
<u>CAUTION</u> Excess iodine may interfere with thyroid function.

Iron      <u>EFFECTS</u> Vital to energy used in red blood cells to carry oxygen. A deficiency causes anemia, with resulting fatigue and sometimes depression.
<u>SOURCES</u> Liver, egg yolks, dried apricots, raisins, fish, beans, legumes, dried fruits—especially apricots and raisins
<u>CAUTION</u> Excess iron can damage organs—especially the liver and heart.

Magnesium      <u>EFFECTS</u> Involved in production of sex hormones. Increases levels of the female hormone progesterone. Helpful for women with PMS.

MINERAL

Magnesium
(cont.)

SOURCES  Soybeans, meat, fish, dairy products, apples, apricots, avocados, bananas, molasses, brown rice, brewer's yeast, figs
CAUTION  Excessive amounts may cause diarrhea.

Manganese

EFFECTS  Helps maintain hormone production. In male laboratory animals, a manganese deficiency causes loss of sex drive, lack of semen, and degeneration of the seminal tubules.
SOURCES  Avocados, nuts, seeds, kelp, whole grains, coffee, tea
CAUTION  Excess doses may cause nerve damage.

Selenium

EFFECTS  A mood booster and energy enhancer. An antioxidant that may slow down the aging process. Helps prevent dandruff and acne. Males need more because of high amount of selenium in sperm.
SOURCES  Brazil nuts, seafood, poultry, organ meats, whole grains, onions, garlic, mushrooms (Selenium content of food is dependent on the extent of its presence in the soil.)
CAUTION  Overdoses can interfere with assimilation of fluoride. Severe overdoses can be toxic.

Zinc

EFFECTS  The "man's mineral"—essential for health of the prostate and for active sperm. A deficiency may cause sexual dysfunction. Even a mild deficiency lowers testosterone levels. (Symptoms of a deficiency: white spots on fingernails, prostate enlargement.)
SOURCES  Pumpkin seeds, oysters, fish, yogurt, legumes, whole grains
CAUTION  Overdoses may interfere with calcium and copper absorption.

# CHAPTER SEVEN

## *Neurotransmitters as Aphrodisiacs*

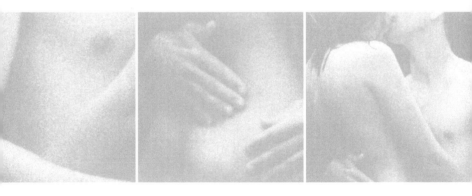

*N*owhere is the power of mind more dramatically demonstrated than in the sexual arena, where erotic thoughts and fantasies routinely arouse desire—even with no external sensory stimulation whatever. The brain is quite capable of inventing and calling into play its own aphrodisiacs—with or without our conscious knowledge.

How does this happen? How can thought—which seemingly has no physical substance—exert such a powerful influence over the body? What is it about the brain that gives it the power to excite us? to move us? to control our bodily processes and even our sex lives? In spite of impressive gains made in brain research, we have only partial answers to these questions. We are just beginning to have the technology available to track thought through the brain, to see the brain in action as it thinks.

## ❧ HOW THE BRAIN INFLUENCES SEX

Although we do not yet have the complete picture of how the brain functions, we know that brain activity produces minute electrical impulses—microvolts—that can be detected by electrodes attached to the scalp and read by an EEG (electroencephalograph). These electrical impulses are fired along the network of nerves, aided in their transit by chemical messengers called *neurotransmitters*.

Neurotransmitters are vital to the communication of messages in the brain's complex networks—including those that control the sex drive. Like the brain itself, neurotransmitters are intimately involved in all aspects of our being—physical, mental, psychological, and emotional. They are only produced in small amounts by the body, but their effects are powerful.

# ❧ THE POWER OF NEUROTRANSMITTERS

The effects of neurotransmitters are widespread and varied—from controlling the sex drive to creating cravings and addictions, affecting emotions and energy levels, and influencing thinking ability and memory. Individual neurotransmitters produce unique effects that sometimes contrast with those of other neurotransmitters.

For example, neurotransmitters can:

- Bring pain or pleasure
- Trigger rage or bring waves of contentment
- Cause depression or create euphoria
- Trigger aggression or stimulate intimacy and bonding

The effects that are produced depend on the individual neurotransmitter involved.

### *The Neurotransmitter/Sex Connection*

Neurotransmitters affect sex both directly and indirectly. They affect sex directly by stimulating or inhibiting sexual arousal and performance, and indirectly by fostering moods, emotions, and even personality traits that either promote or discourage an active, satisfying sex life.

Neurotransmitters are the chemicals in the brain that trigger—or inhibit—the sex drive. They enable the brain to connect the different aspects of sex—physical, psychological, and emotional. Without neurotransmitters we would not enjoy sex or anticipate it with pleasure. We would not be aroused by erotic thoughts and sensations. We would not connect sex with thoughts of love and romance.

### *How Can We Influence Neurotransmitter Levels?*

There is much we can do to achieve optimum neurotransmitter levels and to keep the nervous system operating at peak efficiency. It boils down to the basics of good health—particularly diet and exercise. Neurotransmitter levels can also be favorably influenced by sexual activity, touch, meditation, stress management, and acupuncture. In addition, there are ways to affect specific neurotransmitters, for example by taking certain nutritional supplements.

Of the brain's numerous neurotransmitters, four exert an especially strong influence on sexuality. They are:

- Dopamine
- Serotonin
- Norepinephrine
- Endorphins

All of these neurotransmitters are derived from amino acids found in protein foods. Consequently, diet has a direct connection to neurotransmitter levels that influence sex and is one of the main means by which we can influence them. The following sections include specific suggestions for influencing levels of the major sex-related neurotransmitters.

## ∾ DOPAMINE

Dopamine is the neurotransmitter synonymous with pleasure. It makes us feel good and enables us to enjoy sex and look forward to sexual activity. Dopamine also helps us to perceive and to respond to the sensual messages from our organs of sight, hearing, taste, touch, and smell.

Crucial to sexual arousal, dopamine exerts a strong influence on our emotions and primitive drives, such as sex. It is also partly responsible for muscle movement and for regulating breathing, hunger, and appetite. Dopamine is an excitatory neurotransmitter (one that "excites" neurons to fire). It is stimulating and is a chemical cousin of the amphetamines.

Dopamine is not released continuously. It pulses on and off as it is needed. Each surge brings a positive emotional response. Bliss, ecstasy, euphoria, elation—all are associated with the pulsing of this neurotransmitter through the brain. A powerful surge of dopamine is released at the moment of sexual climax, producing an intense rush of pleasure.

A sudden surge of dopamine is so pleasurable it can be addictive. Part of the reason substances such as cocaine, nicotine, and alcohol are addictive is that they trigger an immediate, major surge of dopamine in the brain, or they raise dopamine levels by causing dopamine to accumulate in the synapses (minute spaces) between cells.

Dopamine is one of the biochemicals responsible for the feelings associated with falling in love, along with its physical signs: flushed skin, heavy breathing, and sweaty palms. The phenomenon of falling in love is so pleasurable that it, too, can be addictive. Those afflicted with this addiction flit from partner to partner, striving to re-experience the thrill of falling in love again. But the novelty of a new partner soon wears off, because the nervous system does not maintain those exhilarating, abnormally high dopamine levels. It protects itself by moderating them. Only a change of partner once again triggers their immoderate release.

Here are some common questions and answers about dopamine and its effects.

## Dopamine: Questions and Answers

*Q. How does dopamine enhance sex?*
Dopamine enhances sex for both men and women by associating sexual activity with pleasure. Dopamine has the following effects:

- Increases the intensity of a sexual experience
- Reinforces sexual desire
- Boosts the sex drive
- Stimulates response to sensual stimuli, such as seductive aromas, romantic music, sensual touching, delicious tastes, erotic images

- Facilitates orgasm
- Increases sexual energy

*Q. How does a dopamine deficiency affect sex?*
Dopamine is a mood enhancer as well as a sex booster. When your dopamine level is too low, both the emotional and physical aspects of your love life suffer. Sensual and seductive messages do not arouse you. Sexual advances from your partner leave you flat. Even when you think about sex, you lack the energy to pursue it. You may have difficulty achieving orgasm. Sex just isn't as much fun anymore.

Sexual aversion is a more extreme condition caused by low dopamine. Individuals with sexual aversion enjoy sex, but only while they are actively engaged in it. Between sexual encounters they do not look forward to having sex. They avoid sexual contact and sexual encounters.

*Q. How does a dopamine deficiency affect the emotions?*
Low dopamine triggers negative emotions and depression, producing an emotional climate hostile to romance. Repeated "firings" of dopamine in the nervous system (such as are produced intentionally by taking drugs) continually stimulate the brain and the emotions. This leads to lowered dopamine levels and emotional exhaustion.

*Q. How does dopamine deficiency affect the mind?*
Low dopamine dulls memory and thinking ability. It can lead to impulsive behavior by affecting a person's ability to plan his or her actions.

*Q. What symptoms may indicate a dopamine deficiency?*
According to Daisy Merey, MD, PhD, the following symptoms might indicate that your dopamine level is too low (or your serotonin level is too high):

- Decreased sex drive
- Fatigue, weakness, or lethargy

- Muscular aches and/or headaches
- Nasal allergies
- Digestive disturbances, such as nausea or constipation
- Increased appetite
- Cravings for caffeine, chocolate, sweets, fat, salt
- Premenstrual breast tenderness in women.

*Q. What are the effects of excess dopamine?*
Although the effects of dopamine are generally pleasurable, you can have too much of a good thing. Excessive dopamine can be too stimulating, resulting in premature ejaculation, or aggravating the problem if it already exists.

Excessive dopamine can also cause problems in personal relationships. When levels of dopamine are too high in the brain's limbic system ("primitive brain") and too low in the cortex ("thinking brain"), the individual may become unsociable and have problems interacting with others. Such an individual is often overly suspicious and prone to bouts of paranoia. Schizophrenia may be related to excessive levels of dopamine in certain areas of the brain. (Most drugs used to treat schizophrenia are designed to lower dopamine levels.)

## How to Boost Your Dopamine Level
Boosting dopamine to normal levels adds zest to sex. Ways to increase dopamine naturally include diet, nutritional supplements, exercise, acupuncture, touching, and having sex. There are also synthetic means of raising dopamine through prescription drugs.

### Diet: High Protein
Dopamine is synthesized in the body from the amino acid tyrosine (also called L-tyrosine). Tyrosine, in turn, can be produced in the body from the amino acid phenylalanine, (also called L-phenylalanine). Both tyrosine and phenylalanine are present in many protein-rich foods, such as:

- Lean red meat
- Chicken
- Turkey
- Seafood
- Tofu
- Beans
- Peas
- Lentils
- Wheat germ
- Seeds
- Nuts

When you need to be alert and want the lift of dopamine, eat protein. A high-protein, low-carbohydrate meal (meat, poultry, or seafood plus salad and green beans) helps raise your dopamine level to keep you mentally alert. Do not eat carbohydrates *before* protein if you need the energizing effects of dopamine. Most protein foods contain both tyrosine and tryptophan, and those two amino acids compete to enter the brain. Carbohydrates work with tryptophan to enable it to enter the brain first, excluding tyrosine. As a result serotonin is produced instead of dopamine. You feel relaxed and content, not alert and energetic.

### *Foods You Crave*

Low dopamine creates cravings for foods and substances that raise dopamine, such as caffeine, chocolate, sweets, fats, and salt. Curiously, one alcoholic drink raises the level of dopamine, while more than one raises the level of serotonin. When you have a craving for caffeine, chocolate, cheese, or salted peanuts, you may be looking for something to raise your level of dopamine—especially if you have other symptoms of low dopamine, such as headache, depression, or fatigue.

*Nutritional Supplements*

Tyrosine and phenylalanine—Supplements of tyrosine and phenylalanine, the nutrients used by the body to synthesize dopamine, are available in health food stores. Tyrosine supplements are often taken to elevate mood, combat depression, suppress appetite, and reduce body fat. Tyrosine has also been used to alleviate symptoms caused by withdrawal from drugs.

Phenylalanine comes in two forms, D-phenylalanine and L-phenylalanine. D-phenylalanine is taken for pain. L-phenylalanine is taken for depression. The two kinds are also sold combined as DLPA.

Both phenylalanine and tyrosine are stimulating to some people and may cause insomnia or anxiety.

Avoid taking either phenylalanine or tyrosine if you are taking antidepressants or an MAO inhibitor, or if you have high blood pressure, phenylketonuria, melanoma skin cancer, or diabetes.

Vitamins and minerals—The synthesis of dopamine in the body is accomplished by enzymatic action, which requires magnesium, iron, inositol, vitamin C, vitamin $B_3$, vitamin $B_6$, and folic acid.

*Exercise*

Exercise has many positive effects for an active, satisfying sex life. In addition to the obvious benefits of producing an attractive, vigorous body and promoting a feeling of well-being, exercise causes beneficial changes in the body's chemistry. It raises glucose levels, which reduces the appetite and increases levels of dopamine and norepinephrine—both of which increase sexual enjoyment and enhance mood.

Physical activity, in general, benefits body, mind, and emotions. Aerobic exercise in particular is a mood elevator and helps build the stamina required for an active sex life. In addition, it promotes the release of endorphins, which make us feel good and mentally alert. To qualify as aerobic, exercise should be nonstop for at least twelve minutes. Ideally, it should involve large, lower-body muscles. Examples are walking, running, dancing, rowing, and cross-country skiing. Sports such as golf, tennis, and football are nonaerobic because they involve stop-and-go activity.

The best exercise is an activity you enjoy, because this increases the chances that you will engage in it readily and regularly. Walking for at least twenty minutes four or more times a week is an example of an aerobic activity that most of us can comfortably accommodate into our schedules.

### Acupuncture

Acupuncture is a technique used in Asian medicine to relieve pain and to heal. It involves the use of sterile, hairlike needles inserted into various parts of the body. Eastern medicine claims that acupuncture relieves pain by releasing blocked energy in the body, allowing it to flow freely once more. Western physicians theorize that acupuncture works because it stimulates release of the pain-killing, pleasure-producing neurotransmitters—dopamine, norepinephrine, and the endorphins.

### Sexual Activity, Touching, and Testosterone

Engaging in sexual activity promotes the release of dopamine, which brings with it a rush of pleasure, thus reinforcing the body-mind association between sex and pleasure. This is also true for touching. A lover's touch or caress triggers a pleasurable release of dopamine.

It is possible that for men, increasing the level of testosterone may also increase the level of dopamine. This is true for animals studied, but it is not yet known if the same holds true for humans.

### Prescription Drugs

Several prescription drugs are used to raise dopamine levels. One, L-dopa, is identical to an amino acid that occurs naturally in the body and is used by the brain in converting tyrosine and phenylalanine to dopamine. L-dopa is prescribed for aging patients whose dopamine levels have significantly decreased. It is often used to treat Parkinson's disease (a dopamine disorder) and depression.

Deprenyl (selegiline) was developed as an antidepressant. It works by stimulating the production of dopamine. Deprenyl is prescribed to restore dopamine to its proper level and to improve brain functioning. It is said to repair damaged brain cells, stimulate memory, and improve learning ability.

Wellbutrin (bupropion) is prescribed to combat depression and help restore the sex drive—unlike other antidepressants, which often suppress the sex drive. Wellbutrin supposedly works by boosting the activity of dopamine receptors in the brain.

*Dopamine and Addictive Substances*

Although the release of dopamine is pleasurable, it is not always beneficial. It may be triggered by a harmful substance. The rush of pleasure that accompanies a surge of dopamine can "reward" a destructive addiction. Cocaine addiction is one example. Cocaine affects nerve cells in the brain that trigger a release of dopamine. Dopamine carries its pleasurable message throughout the pathways of the nervous system, essentially saying, "Cocaine brings pleasure." Strong stimulants such as cocaine and amphetamines, besides being dangerous in other ways, are ultimately harmful to the brain and endocrine system because they cause an immediate overproduction of dopamine followed by its sharp depletion. Such a severe drop in dopamine can cause memory blackouts and can adversely affect the ability to think clearly.

## ∾ SEROTONIN

Serotonin is dopamine's opposite. When tension, worry, or anxiety make for sleepless nights, when you are too tired or depressed to think about having sex, serotonin can come to the rescue. Serotonin fights depression and anxiety and makes us feel safe and fulfilled. It promotes a more relaxed state along with the ability to get much-needed sleep. (On the other hand, when sleep is not a problem and what you are looking for is more sexual energy, more serotonin is not the answer. Instead, you will need to avoid serotonin boosters, such as high-carbohydrate foods, especially before having sex.)

Serotonin works more slowly and regularly than dopamine. Dopamine's effect is direct, immediate, and stimulating. But dopamine is not always active—it surges on an "as needed" basis. In contrast to dopamine's surges, serotonin's output is steady, slow, and rhythmic.

Serotonin is self-regulating. It not only regulates dopamine levels but its own level, slowing or speeding up its rhythmic pulsation as needed. Even though serotonin often opposes the effects of dopamine, it, too, is needed for an active sex life. Like dopamine, serotonin makes us feel good—but in a different way. Serotonin's effects can be summed up in four "s-words": Serotonin is soothing and sleep-inducing, making us feel safe and secure.

## Serotonin: Questions and Answers

*Q. How does serotonin enhance sex?*
Serotonin normally tones down the aggressive sex drive and any sexual excesses brought on by dopamine. However, serotonin is a complex neurotransmitter. It has multiple receptors, some of which discourage sex while others, under certain chemical circumstances, directly stimulate sexual activity.

Serotonin enhances sex primarily in several ways. It:

- Plays a critical role in controlling negative emotions and removing tension and anxiety that can inhibit sexual arousal

- Promotes sexual responsiveness

- Creates optimism and other positive emotional states conducive to enjoying sex
- Facilitates warmth and intimacy
- Fights depression
- Helps prevent premature ejaculation by delaying orgasm
- Promotes selectivity in choosing a sexual partner and defuses impulsive sexual arousal

*Q. What happens if you have too little serotonin?*
In general, low serotonin produces conditions that affect sex adversely, primarily by triggering negative emotions. There is one positive effect, however: Abnormally low serotonin increases sexual responsiveness. Both men and women with low serotonin levels reach orgasm more quickly.

A depleted serotonin level can trigger antisocial behavior, including violence and aggressive, abusive sex. One function of serotonin is to enable us to keep anger and aggression under control. Serotonin depletion makes it hard to put on the emotional brakes.

Based on animal studies, it is thought that low serotonin may be implicated in overly aggressive sexual behavior. Animals whose serotonin was lowered engaged in a sexual frenzy. They became indiscriminate in their sexual behavior, mounting both males and females and animals of different species. They even mounted dead animals. During sex they wounded, tortured, killed, and even devoured their mates. Female rats whose serotonin level was lowered behaved sexually like males. They mounted smaller males and other females.

In *The Alchemy of Love and Lust*, Theresa L. Crenshaw, MD, raises some intriguing questions based on these animal studies: Could violent sex offenders have neurotransmitter disorders that cause their aggression? Could their violence be controlled by medications that increase serotonin, medications such as Prozac? From what we know about the powerful impact of neurotransmitters on the emotions, this might be an area well worth investigating.

Daisy Merey, MD, PhD, an authority on the connection between neurotransmitters and weight control, feels that dopamine and serotonin are the prime regulators of our health and well-being. We are only beginning to find out exactly how powerful they are. As Dr. Merey puts it, "What we know about neurotransmitters is just the tip of the iceberg. More and more studies are showing the significance of neurotransmitters, not just for our health but for the way we behave. Anger, restlessness, sexual desire, obesity, anxiety, depression—neurotransmitters are involved with them all."

*Q. What are the symptoms of a serotonin deficiency?*
According to Dr. Merey, a serotonin deficiency can keep us from feeling full and can cause us to overeat. In addition, low serotonin (or excess dopamine) causes:

- Feelings of uneasiness
- Anxiety
- Irritability
- Anger
- Restlessness
- Insomnia
- Breast tenderness and other PMS-like symptoms for women, even when they do not have PMS
- Slow or reduced flow of urine
- Increased body temperature
- Diarrhea, irritable bowel syndrome
- Racing heart
- Increased blood pressure

- Cravings for carbohydrates
- Cravings for alcohol and smoking

*Q. What are the effects of excessive serotonin?*

- May temporarily heighten sexual response. Initially, serotonin removes stress and anxiety, which may heighten sexual response. However, the body soon adjusts itself to these higher serotonin levels and the anxiety returns.

- Prevents premature ejaculation. High serotonin delays orgasm and thus can prevent premature ejaculation. In fact, Prozac (which raises serotonin levels) was the first drug used successfully to treat premature ejaculation.

- Deflates the sex drive. High serotonin levels can be so calming they inhibit sexual stimulation and arousal. They deflate the sex drive and the ability to achieve orgasm. This also occurs when serotonin levels are raised artificially by antidepressant drugs such as Prozac.

- Flattens emotional response. Although high serotonin levels make some individuals slightly euphoric, they make others feel emotionally anesthetized. While this emotional flattening may help those in the depths of depression, it effectively takes the spice out of life and the thrill out of sex.

*Q. How does serotonin affect appetite and weight?*

Low serotonin increases our appetite and causes us to crave substances that will raise our serotonin, for example, sugar, alcohol, bread, bagels, pasta, and potato chips. The combination of increased appetite plus cravings for sugar, alcohol, and starchy foods is a recipe for weight gain.

Sugar cravings and weight gain are more likely to occur in women than in men because estrogen affects serotonin levels. Falling estrogen levels are thought to cause lowered serotonin, which triggers appetite and cravings for sugar and carbohydrates.

*Q. How does serotonin affect sleep?*

Serotonin, along with the amino acid tryptophan, is a precursor to melatonin, a hormone that regulates the body's internal clock and affects sleep patterns. Low levels of serotonin can make falling asleep difficult, if not impossible.

## How to Raise Your Serotonin Level

*Diet and Nutritional Supplements*

Tryptophan—What you eat has a direct and immediate impact on your serotonin levels. In order for your body to synthesize serotonin it must have the amino acid tryptophan (also called L-tryptophan). This amino acid occurs naturally in such foods as turkey, red meat, chicken, sunflower seeds, nuts, and bananas. Tryptophan used to be available as a nutritional supplement and was sold in health food stores. In 1989 a batch contaminated with bacteria forced the removal of all tryptophan from the market. Before its removal tryptophan was widely used to treat depression and insomnia. Today a modified form of tryptophan called 5HTP (5-hydroxy-L-tryptophan) is available in health food stores. It is described below.

Carbohydrates—Since tryptophan needs carbohydrates in order to be absorbed by the brain, its effects are heightened when tryptophan-rich foods are eaten along with high-carbohydrate foods such as bread, potatoes, cereal, fruit, and corn. What happens when you eat a typical dinner of meat and potatoes, with some bread or corn? The resulting combination of tryptophan and carbohydrates causes your serotonin level to rise. You feel relaxed, content, secure. You may even doze off.

When you feel anxious, edgy, irritable, or can't sleep, do you find yourself craving a bagel, potato chips, a drink—anything that will raise your serotonin level? An efficient way to increase serotonin is to eat a carbohydrate food first and then a food rich in tryptophan, such as turkey. The carbohydrates enable tryptophan to enter the brain before tyrosine (also in protein foods, but a dopamine stimulator). Since the amino acids compete for entry into the brain, only one can enter. With the help of carbohydrates, tryptophan wins and tyrosine is excluded.

Melatonin—Melatonin is a popular nonprescription supplement used primarily to relieve insomnia, jet lag, and depression. It is actually a hormone whose function is to regulate the body's internal clock, or sleeping–waking cycle. Melatonin is thought to be strongly connected to the release of serotonin. Taking melatonin supplements would thus increase serotonin levels.

5HTP—In the brain, tryptophan is first converted into 5HTP (hydroxytryptophan) by an enzyme. The 5HTP then crosses the blood-brain barrier and is converted to serotonin. Supplements of 5HTP are available. Since it is a serotonin precursor, 5HTP raises serotonin levels and is said to control appetite and the food cravings triggered by low serotonin.

Herbs—The herbal supplements St. John's wort and ginkgo biloba decrease the reabsorption of serotonin by transmitting nerve cells. The result is that serotonin accumulates in the gaps between nerve cells and serotonin levels rise. St. John's wort is a natural antidepressant. Ginkgo is taken for many reasons, but primarily to increase memory and mental acuity. (See Chapter 3, "Herbs as Aphrodisiacs," for more on St. John's wort and ginkgo biloba.)

*Weight Gain*

Gaining excess weight raises serotonin. Needless to say, there are healthier ways to raise serotonin. (Even taking a bath, rubbing velvet on your cheek, looking at a photograph of your family or your pet—whatever makes you feel content or protected—raises your serotonin level.)

Serotonin is involved with insulin, a hormone that helps the body use sugar. Diabetes, a disease in which there is insufficient insulin or the body cannot use it properly, causes weight gain. This in turn raises the serotonin level. This becomes a vicious cycle because obesity itself increases serotonin, sometimes to the point of inducing lethargy and lowering the sex drive.

*Prescription Drugs*
Certain antidepressant prescription drugs work by raising serotonin levels. Two examples are Prozac and Zoloft. However, even though such drugs may alleviate anxiety, they may also flatten emotional response, making it difficult to achieve arousal or orgasm.

## *How to Lower Your Serotonin Level*

*Diet*
When you want to be mentally alert and feel energized, what you need is lower serotonin and higher dopamine. In order to achieve this, eat protein *before* eating carbohydrates to allow tyrosine to enter the brain instead of tryptophan. Better yet, hold off on the carbohydrates until you are ready to relax.

*Nutritional Supplements*
Serotonin levels can also be lowered by taking supplements of other amino acids (besides tyrosine) that compete with tryptophan for entry into the brain. Weight trainers do this to prevent the fatigue caused by rising levels of tryptophan (and hence serotonin) as their muscles use up other available amino acids. To lower serotonin, weight trainers take supplements of branched-chain amino acids (BCAAs). BCAAs are made up of the three amino acids leucine, isoleucine, and valine. During a weight-lifting session, BCAAs are broken down and burned up for energy. As BCAAs are depleted, tryptophan levels rise—with a consequent rise in serotonin. Serotonin creates fatigue. In order to prevent this, the weight trainers take supplemental BCAAs before their workout. The BCAAs overwhelm tryptophan and prevent it from crossing the blood-brain barrier to make serotonin. The result—increased endurance.

Norepinephrine (or noradrenaline) is chemically similar to dopamine and, like dopamine, is both a sex-booster and mood-enhancer. Both are synthesized in the brain from the same amino acids, phenylalanine and tyrosine, and each can be chemically converted to the other in the brain.

Norepinephrine is an excitatory neurotransmitter, meaning it excites neurons (nerve cells) to fire. It also excites us. Norepinephrine motivates us and incites us to action. It helps us view life positively and with zest, and plays an important role in our reaction to stress and in the normal functioning of our immune system.

Norepinephrine boosts memory, learning, and our ability to pay attention and stay focused on a task. It also sends messages to endocrine glands causing them to release hormones. It is a super-neurotransmitter—one of the most important neurotransmitters in the brain.

## Norepinephrine: Questions and Answers

*Q. How does norepinephrine enhance sex?*
Norepinephrine enhances sex directly by boosting the sex drive and indirectly by promoting emotional states conducive to love-making. It is the primary neurotransmitter used by the nervous system to increase sexual interest and activity. In addition, norepinephrine:

- Helps regulate sexual behavior
- Stimulates the release of hormones that regulate fertility, the sex drive, appetite, and metabolism
- Generates positive moods and emotions conducive to lovemaking

*Q. What happens if you have too little norepinephrine?*
Depression—Norepinephrine, along with dopamine, is motivational. It promotes a zest for living. When norepinephrine

levels fall, the result can be apathy, lethargy, depression. Some drugs used to treat depression—tricyclic antidepressants—work by causing an increase in norepinephrine levels.

Magnifies effects of stress—Norepinephrine is depleted in states of chronic stress. This norepinephrine deficiency contributes to the harmful effects of stress.

Affects immune system—Norepinephrine is involved in the release of growth hormone, which is needed for proper functioning of the immune system. Depleted norepinephrine levels can lower the body's resistance to infections, autoimmune diseases, and cancer.

*Q. What happens if your norepinephrine level is too high?*
An excess of norepinephrine (like a deficiency of serotonin) can lead to irritability and outbursts of rage.

### How to Raise Your Norepinephrine Level
Dopamine and norepinephrine are so similar chemically that what affects one usually affects the other. Thus the recommendations for dopamine concerning nutrition, exercise, and so on hold true for norepinephrine.

*Nutrition*
Like dopamine, norepinephrine is synthesized in the body from the amino acids tyrosine and phenylalanine. Thus, the nutritional principles for increasing dopamine also apply to norepinephrine.

Protein-rich foods—Researchers at the Massachusetts Institute of Technology demonstrated that levels of norepinephrine can rise after a *single* protein-rich meal. Foods that boost norepinephrine include:

- Lean red meat
- Chicken
- Turkey
- Seafood
- Tofu

- Beans
- Peas
- Lentils

Nutritional supplements—The nutritional supplement tyrosine (also called L-tyrosine) boosts norepinephrine because tyrosine is used by the body to synthesize norepinephrine. The supplement DLPA (an abbreviation for the two forms of phenylalanine: D-phenylalanine and L-phenylalanine) is the suggested way to take supplemental phenylalanine, which, like tyrosine, is a precursor of norepinephrine.

Both phenylalanine and tyrosine are stimulating to some people and may cause insomnia or anxiety.

Avoid taking either phenylalanine or tyrosine if you are taking antidepressants or an MAO inhibitor, or if you have high blood pressure, phenylketonuria, melanoma skin cancer, or diabetes.

*Exercise*

As with dopamine, exercise helps boost norepinephrine. Aerobic exercise in particular helps to normalize both low and high levels of norepinephrine. By enhancing the body's ability to deal with stress, exercise helps prevent the depletion of norepinephrine.

*Acupuncture*

Like dopamine, the release of norepinephrine is stimulated by acupuncture therapy.

*Temperature*

Higher temperatures can affect neurotransmitter levels, especially those of norepinephrine. Higher temperatures are stimulating to the brain; cooler temperatures are relaxing. Higher temperatures thus raise levels of the stimulating neurotransmitter norepinephrine, while cooler temperatures are more favorable to raising serotonin.

# ～ ENDORPHINS

Endorphins are small protein substances recently discovered in the brain. They are opiate-like chemicals whose effects are like those of the neurotransmitters, although technically, endorphins are not neurotransmitters. Some call them polypeptides; others call them neurohormones. In any case, endorphins are chemical messengers related in function to both neurotransmitters and hormones.

Endorphins, like dopamine, are the bringers of pleasure. They are also the killers of pain, the body's natural morphine. In fact, the word *endorphin* is derived from *endogenous* and *morphine*, meaning "morphine from within."

Endorphins first came to public attention in connection with the "runner's high." This natural high is triggered during intense aerobic exercise and is caused by a rise in endorphins (and dopamine), which replaces the physical pain of the runner with elation, optimism, and a feeling of well-being that continue after the exercise has ended. It is a well-known phenomenon that runners and joggers can become addicted to their endorphin high to the point of compulsively engaging in that activity.

Endorphins and dopamine work together. Endorphins are used by the brain to lessen sensitivity to pain and open the dopamine pathways to pleasure. Endorphins are the body's own tranquilizers. Chemically, they are very similar to morphine. They even bind to the same kind of receptors in the brain. Endorphins are also chemically similar to heroin, and operate in much the same way. They both replace pain with euphoria. Heroin's effects last longer because endorphins, although very powerful, are released as a temporary measure to protect us from the immediate pain of an injury or a stressful situation.

The stimulus for endorphin release does not have to be painful. Listening to beautiful music, touching your partner, floating in a float tank—all these are examples of pleasurable stimuli that cause the release of endorphins.

### How Do Endorphins Enhance Sex?

Endorphins stimulate sex by raising the level of dopamine, which boosts the sex drive and brings waves of pleasure. When endorphins are released, they open up the dopamine pathways, allowing more dopamine to flow through.

Endorphins are awakened by the sense of touch. When lovers hold each other in their arms, their endorphin levels begin to rise. The lovers are flushed with pleasure and contentment. Endorphins reward the lovers' physical contact with intense pleasure, which leads—not surprisingly—to more touching.

Endorphins also induce emotional states that are conducive to sex. Endorphins relieve anxiety and stress to clear the way for sexual pleasure. They are the brain's natural tranquilizers as well as its analgesics, or painkillers.

An important function of the endorphins is to combat the effects of extreme stress, whether it be physical or psychological. Needless to say, stress is the enemy of pleasure and of the capacity to enjoy sex. By combating stress, endorphins affect mood and often relieve depression.

Endorphins work in their painkilling capacity to anaesthetize pain that might interfere with sexual enjoyment, replacing pain with pleasure. When pain and discomfort are held in check during sex, it is due to the anesthetizing power of the endorphins.

### How to Increase Your Level of Endorphins

Endorphins are released in response to physical stimuli. They are also released in response to thoughts and emotions. Exercise, touching, acupuncture, and even the fiery pain ignited by biting into a hot chili pepper—all these release endorphins. So does the mind. The mind's ability to generate endorphin production probably accounts for the pain-relieving effect of placebos. Placebos relieve pain because patients *believe* they are taking a painkiller. Although the placebo effect is produced unconsciously, endorphins can also be increased by conscious thought. Endorphin levels can be raised with mind/body exercises and biofeedback. Thus you can enlist both your body and your mind to encourage the release of endorphins.

*Exercise*
Exercise increases endorphins, which is one of the reasons exercise relieves stress and elevates mood. Aerobic exercise is the best kind for relieving stress. To be aerobic, an activity must keep the heart pumping at an elevated level for at least twelve minutes. Running, jogging, skiing, dancing, and walking are some examples, because they involve continued movement of the large body muscles. Sports that involve stop-and-go activity, such as golf, tennis, and basketball, are nonaerobic. This is not to imply that nonaerobic exercise is not beneficial, too—it is just that aerobic exercise is more apt to reduce stress by raising endorphin levels.

*Laugh, Smile, Think Positive!*
Norman Cousins, who used laughter and the power of the mind to recover from life-threatening illness, said that ten minutes of belly laughter can result in two hours of pain-free sleep. Indeed, laughter stimulates the release of painkilling, mood-lifting endorphins.

Smiling may also raise endorphin levels. *In The Alchemy of Love and Lust*, Theresa L. Crenshaw, MD, notes that some psychologists and neurologists believe that smiling and other facial movements momentarily divert blood from the brain to the face. This changes brain temperature, stimulating the brain's synthesis of endorphins.

By the same token, thinking positive thoughts raises endorphin levels. This may be why positive thinking really can make you feel better. As your endorphin levels rise, so does your mood.

# CHAPTER EIGHT

## *Hormones as Aphrodisiacs*

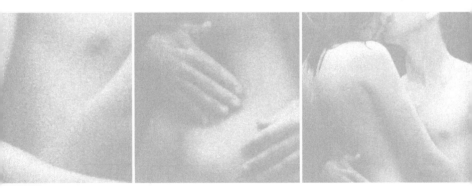

*T*hroughout life our sexuality is controlled by hormones. Even before birth, hormones are at work controlling our sexual development. It is the chemistry of hormones that directs the development of our sexual organs and later our secondary sexual characteristics such as beard growth in men and breast development in women. Hormones instigate and regulate the menstrual cycle. They create the peaks and valleys of our sexual desire. They arouse. They depress. Hormones can precipitate aggressive or receptive sexual behavior. They are the force behind the sex drive, the prime instigator and controller of sexual desire. In many respects, the chemistry of love begins with the chemistry of hormones.

## ❧ THE POWER OF HORMONES

What are hormones? Why do they exert such a powerful control over our lives and our sexuality? How can we tap their power to enhance sex and boost our sex drive? Hormones are chemical messengers that come primarily from the endocrine glands. They enable the endocrine system to regulate activity in other cells and organs of the body. Endocrine glands pour secretions directly into the bloodstream. Examples include the sex glands (ovaries and testes), the pituitary gland, and the thyroid. (Exocrine glands, on the other hand, do not secrete into the bloodstream and do not produce hormones. The salivary glands, sweat glands, and tear glands are examples of exocrine glands.)

Hormones are considered messengers because they enable a gland to control activity of a cell or organ from a distance. For example, when a female reaches puberty, her ovaries release sex hormones. These ovarian hormones trigger activity in other parts of the body, such as the development of the breasts, broadening of the hips, and growth of underarm hair.

### How Do Hormones Work?

In simple terms, this is how a hormone transmission takes place: a gland secretes a hormone into the bloodstream. The hormone is programmed for a specific target—a cell or organ that the gland regulates. Once released, the hormone circulates in the blood until it is picked up by a receptor cell on its target. When contact is made, the hormone binds to the receptor, thus delivering its message—a message that triggers a reaction in the target tissue.

The word *hormone* comes from the Greek *hormon*, meaning "to excite or arouse," which is an apt description of what happens when a hormone delivers its message: The target tissue is aroused to activity. Its reaction may be immediate and of short duration or it may be more long-lasting. Hormones are very powerful and therefore are released only in minute amounts. Even slight fluctuations in hormone levels can affect the body, mind, or emotions.

### Kinds of Hormones

Hormones are classified in two groups, based on their chemical structure:

- Steroids
- Peptides

Steroids are made from cholesterol and have a characteristic four-ring structure. Sex hormones are steroids. The male hormones are called *androgens*, of which *testosterone* is the most active. The female hormones are the estrogens and progesterone. In addition, DHEA (dehydroepiandrosterone), which is part of the androgen family, is an important sex hormone precursor that can be converted to the other sex hormones. (A precursor is a substance that turns into another or more active substance. DHEA, for example, can be used by the body to make testosterone and other androgens and to make estrogens.)

The androgens, or male hormones, appear to be responsible for sexual arousal. They affect both the endocrine system, which produces hormones, and the nervous system, which governs the mind and the emotions. Women produce androgens, but in smaller amounts. These small amounts are essential for maintaining normal sexual desire in women.

The other group of hormones, peptides, are made up of amino acids strung together in chains. Gastrointestinal hormones and the pituitary hormone oxytocin are examples of peptides, or protein-derived, hormones. Oxytocin is connected to sex, love, and romance: it is stimulated by touching and makes us feel good—which stimulates more touching. In both its responsiveness to touch and its mood-elevating properties, oxytocin is similar to endorphins. Oxytocin promotes feelings of warmth, intimacy, and bonding and is thus a powerful adjunct to sexual love, even though it does not stimulate the sex drive by itself. Oxytocin is also involved in reproduction, as it produces contractions of the uterus during labor and stimulates milk flow in breastfeeding women.

## Chemical Cousins of Hormones

### Neurotransmitters

The sexual power of hormones is similar to the sexual power of neurotransmitters. They are chemical cousins. In fact, some hormones can be neurotransmitters and vice versa. Norepinephrine is an example. When it is produced by nerve cells and travels through nerve pathways it is a neurotransmitter; when it is produced by the adrenal glands and travels through the bloodstream it is a hormone.

### Pheromones

Hormones have another group of chemical relatives: pheromones. Sex hormones are the "parents," or source, of male and female pheromones. Hormones spawn pheromones in two ways. First, it is the rising levels of sex hormones at puberty that initiate pheromone production. Second, hormones supply the chemical building blocks of pheromones. Pheromones are produced from the byproducts of sex hormones that are broken down by the actions of enzymes and skin bacteria. For instance, the male pheromones androstenol and androstenone are derived from the male hormone testosterone or its precursor, DHEA. The female hormones progesterone and the estrogens also produce chemicals that are thought to be pheromones.

## ❧ HORMONES AND THE HUMAN SEX DRIVE

As with all mammals, the human sex drive is hormone-driven. However, our sex drive differs in one important respect from that of other mammals. Most female mammals become sexually receptive and mate only during estrus, or heat, at certain times of the year. Their heat periods coincide with ovulation, which maximizes the chances for pregnancy. Human females, on the other hand, can enjoy sexual intercourse at any stage of their monthly ovulatory cycle, as well as after removal of the ovaries or following menopause. Unlike other mammals, ovulation in human females is not marked by a change in behavior or other signs obvious to males. Consequently, neither the male nor female can determine if she is capable of conceiving on any particular day. In humans the sex drive is not irrevocably linked to the probability of initiating a pregnancy. The sex drive is not merely for propagation of the species.

### How Shifting Hormone Levels Affect Relationships
When a woman is not ovulating, her sex drive is still there, but it does fluctuate. It rises and falls along with the rise and fall of an individual's sex hormones. This is true for both men and women. Shifting hormone levels directly impact the sex drive and can wreak havoc in a relationship if we do not recognize or understand what is happening. As hormone levels rise and

fall, so does sexual interest. It is as natural as the rise and fall of the tides, as predictable as the cycle of the seasons. The problem is that we do not realize what is happening because we do not understand body chemistry. When sex loses its zest, we tend to blame our partner or ourselves. In many cases we should blame it on our hormones.

## How Aging Affects Hormone Levels

Hormone levels are constantly changing—throughout the day, week, and month, and, eventually, over the years. Between the ages of twenty-five and thirty our hormone levels are at their peak. Then, led by DHEA, they begin to decline. (DHEA declines at the rate of about 2 percent a year.)

When this decline begins, we do not notice the change. It is when we reach middle age that it hits us. We can't do the things we used to do. We're not as strong as we once were. We become tired more easily. Our sex drive has diminished. Many things we used to enjoy now seem like too much effort. We are getting flabby, maybe fat, in spite of our efforts to exercise or diet.

When menopause strikes, women are hit even harder. For women, the hormonal decline now accelerates. It is much more precipitous than anything men will experience. The effect of this hormonal loss on a woman's sex life can be severe. In addition to emotional distress, hormonal depletion can decrease sexual desire and arousal. It causes vaginal dryness and thinning of the vaginal lining, which makes intercourse painful. It can cause bladder problems. As Katherine Hepburn is credited with saying, "Old age is not for sissies!"

Is this decline inevitable? Perhaps not.

## Can We Control Our Hormone Levels?

When hormones reach their peak, we hit our prime. As they decline, they bring on the symptoms of aging. Hormones obviously exert a tremendous influence on our lives, but we do have some control over them.

## Diet and Nutritional Supplements

Since the body does not store hormones to any great extent, they are continually being replenished and produced. This gives us a chance to step in and affect hormone levels favorably. Since hormones are synthesized by the body from substances obtained from food, we can increase hormone levels by what we eat and by taking nutritional supplements. (See the discussions of individual hormones that follow for the foods and supplements to take.)

## Stress Reduction

Hormone levels are directly influenced by stress—both physical and emotional. By introducing stress-reducing strategies into your life, you can bring hormone levels into balance. Exercise and meditation are examples of two natural stress-relieving strategies. Having sex is another. In addition to relieving stress, sex increases levels of sex hormones. This leads to the desire for more sexual activity. "Use it or lose it."

## Exercise

Regular exercise equals better sex. There is a definite connection between being physically active and sustaining an energetic sex life. Just as exercise boosts sex, stopping a regular exercise routine can cause a noticeable decline in the sex drive.

Why does exercise enhance sex? In addition to increasing strength and energy and reducing stress, regular exercise raises testosterone levels in both men and women. The sex drive is testosterone-driven. Exercise also improves the functioning of the cardiovascular system, which aids men in having an erection and helps prevent impotence. Thus exercise helps give us the strength and energy for sex, counteracts stress that can inhibit sex, improves cardiovascular function necessary for male performance, and boosts hormonal levels that stimulate sexual activity.

*Positive Thinking*

Hormone levels are affected not only by what we do, but by what we think. Positive thoughts raise hormone levels. Negative thoughts decrease them. Positive (or negative) thinking can control hormones.

*Hormone Supplementation*

If medical intervention is required, physicians can prescribe natural or synthetic hormone boosters. Some hormone supplements are made from phytochemicals (plant chemicals) and are available in health food stores. They come in several different forms, such as tablets, pills, creams, and suppositories. In the sections below on testosterone, estrogen, progesterone, DHEA, and in the interview with Dr. Merey I will discuss how to supplement individual hormones.

## ∾ TESTOSTERONE

Testosterone is the most active of the male sex hormones, or androgens. It is the primary male hormone, the one that controls male sexual development and the sex drive. Outside the sexual arena, testosterone influences the male's overall physical health and emotional outlook.

There are two common myths about testosterone. One is that it is an exclusively male hormone. It is not, although males produce a much greater amount of it than females. The other is that testosterone is the only hormone that affects the sex drive. This is not true either, though its effect on sex exceeds that of the other hormones, in both men and women. What is true about testosterone is that it is *the* hormone that directs male development and sexuality. For men it is the hormone of strength, sex, and stamina. For both sexes testosterone is nature's ultimate aphrodisiac, the hormone responsible for the sex drive and sexual desire.

### Testosterone: Questions and Answers

*Q. How does testosterone affect men?*

Testosterone keeps men feeling sexy, strong, healthy, self-confident, and assertive. It holds at bay the symptoms commonly associated with aging.

In the adult male, testosterone:

- Controls the sex drive
- Is necessary for sexual arousal
- Increases sexual fantasies
- Controls sperm production
- Controls ability to maintain an erection
- Builds muscle mass
- Raises metabolism to burn fat
- Elevates mood
- Boosts confidence
- Supplies drive and ambition
- Increases assertive behavior
- Improves memory
- Helps prevent osteoporosis
- Lowers cholesterol
- Protects against heart disease

*Q. What are the effects of excessive testosterone?*

Normally, testosterone produces optimism, self-confidence, competitiveness, and assertive behavior—qualities often thought of as positive for success. Excessive testosterone, however, can escalate these qualities to destructive and dangerous extremes. It can make a person:

- Domineering, controlling, power-hungry
- Overly aggressive, abusive, violent

- Irritable, ill-tempered, unpleasant, angry
- Overly competitive, intolerant of defeat
- Irresponsible, impetuous, unreliable
- Unsympathetic, inconsiderate, disrespectful, boorish

*Q. What are the symptoms of low testosterone?*
Sexual problems—A lack of libido, or sexual desire, is one of the most commonly reported symptoms of a low testosterone level. This is not the same thing as impotence, in which sexual desire may be present but the ability to maintain an erection is not. A man low in testosterone may be physically capable of having sex but has little or no interest in initiating sexual activity. He may feel impotent even though he is not.

In addition to a decrease in libido, low testosterone can cause a decreased volume of ejaculatory fluid.

Health problems—A deficiency of testosterone accelerates the aging process. Symptoms of low testosterone include a feeling of general malaise, loss of vitality, and various signs associated with aging:

- Lessening of strength and muscle mass
- Increase in fat and flabbiness
- Decrease in bone mass
- Diminished flexibility and mobility
- Anemia
- The appearance of having aged prematurely

Emotional problems—Low testosterone can cause depression and apathy, a decrease in a zest for living, and lack of interest in activities that were once enjoyable. Also, low testosterone can be responsible for a low level of drive or ambition.

*Q. Does a man's testosterone level fluctuate?*
A man's testosterone level is not consistent. It has ups and downs, cycling every 15 to 20 minutes. It fluctuates with the

time of day and even with the seasons. (One study found that testosterone peaks in December.) Testosterone is highest in the morning on first awakening. During the day it may fall by as much as one-third to one-half. These constant fluctuations in testosterone level make it difficult to get an accurate reading on an individual's testosterone level.

One study was conducted to see if there is any difference in testosterone levels among men of different occupations. The study included ninety-two men in eight occupations, plus an unemployed category. For the occupations studied, ministers had the lowest testosterone levels; professional football players and actors had the highest. Trial lawyers scored higher in testosterone than did non-trial lawyers.

*Q. What is a "normal" testosterone level?*
There is a wide range of testosterone levels that are all considered normal. This means that a man can have a "normal" level of testosterone even after his testosterone level has declined with aging. For example, a man who has a "high normal" level of testosterone at his peak may still have more testosterone in later years, after his testosterone has declined, than a man still at his peak whose testosterone is in the "low normal" range. Nevertheless, about one-third of all men experience a mid-life drop in testosterone significant enough to affect the body and emotions. By age 65, more than 60 percent of all men have low levels of testosterone, even though only about 30 percent of them fall below the "normal" range.

*Q. Is the strength of your sex drive determined by your testosterone level?*
Recent research indicates that it is not. It appears that for both men and women there is a minimum amount of testosterone needed to switch on sexual desire. This "switch-on" level seems to vary among individuals. We might assume that additional testosterone above that level would increase sexual desire, but this is not the case. More testosterone above the

"switch-on" amount does not boost sexual desire or the amount of sexual activity. On the other hand, lowered testosterone levels diminish the sex drive eventually (but not immediately) for both men and women.

Sex drive is determined by a number of factors, not by testosterone alone. There is no evidence that testosterone is solely responsible for variations in the sex drive between individuals, male or female. Other factors, including other hormones, play a role in determining the strength of sexual desire. Similarly, there is no evidence that an individual's testosterone level affects his or her sexual orientation.

*Q. How much testosterone do women produce?*
Women produce about 0.2 mg of testosterone a day—about 5 to 10 percent of the amount men do. Of this amount, about half is produced by the ovaries and adrenal glands. The remaining half is synthesized from hormone precursors, such as DHEA. As with a man, a woman's testosterone production declines with age, but far more rapidly. By the time she is 40, a woman's testosterone level is only half of what it was when she was twenty. Many women are deficient in testosterone by the time they reach menopause. The decline in testosterone varies from woman to woman along with the severity of symptoms from testosterone loss.

*Q. What does testosterone do for women?*
It is the small amount of testosterone normally produced by women that gives them their sexual desire, or libido. Testosterone also helps relieve menopausal symptoms, restores energy, strengthens bones, and relieves depression. Although women produce only a fraction of the testosterone that men do, this does not mean that they only have a fraction of the sex drive of a man. Rather, women have a greater sensitivity to testosterone than men do—they respond to much smaller amounts of the hormone.

Testosterone helps make women sexually receptive, because testosterone receptors in the nipples, clitoris, and vagina make these areas sensitive to sexual stimulation.

*Q. How does a deficiency in testosterone affect women?*
Susan Rako, MD, has identified a condition she calls "female androgen deficiency syndrome." This deficiency makes sex less enjoyable and makes it more difficult to reach orgasm. In addition, a testosterone deficiency is often accompanied by a low energy level.

A woman's testosterone level declines naturally as a result of menopause, including artificially induced menopause, hysterectomy. For some women, this decline in testosterone leads to depression, fatigue, headaches, reduced sexual desire, reduced muscle mass, thinning pubic hair, and memory loss.

Testosterone affects a woman's sexual response because without testosterone a woman loses sensitivity to sexual pleasure in her nipples and genitals and consequently becomes less sensitive to sexual stimulation.

## How to Affect Testosterone Levels

*Diet and Nutritional Supplements*
Zinc—Unlike neurotransmitters, hormones are not protein-based chemicals and therefore are not synthesized by the body from the proteins we eat. The only single nutrient linked to testosterone is zinc, which is needed in order to produce DHT (dihydroxytestosterone), a testosterone enzyme. Zinc is stored in the testes and is needed for normal sexual functioning of men. Oysters are the richest natural source of zinc, which may explain their reputation as an aphrodisiac. Other rich sources are pumpkin seeds, sunflower seeds, seafood, organ meats, mushrooms, wheat germ, and brewer's yeast.

Dieting—Obesity affects testosterone levels because fat produces its own estrogen, the principal female hormone.

Although an obese man's elevated estrogen levels do not cause feminization, they can cause testosterone to be excreted rather than retained. Thus elevated estrogen levels caused by obesity can lead to diminished testosterone levels.

Alcohol for women?—It has been found that alcohol triggers women to produce more testosterone. The same is not true for men. It has been speculated that this increase in testosterone may be why women who have been drinking alcohol may seem more sexually approachable, or more sexually aggressive.

DHEA supplementation—DHEA is a hormone precursor that can be converted by the body to whatever sex hormone is needed. It is part of the androgen family and is most often converted to testosterone, which helps explain the claims for vitality, weight loss, and increased libido made for it. DHEA is sold over the counter. Suggested doses are usually 25 mg for women and 50 mg for men. DHEA is discussed in more detail later in this chapter.

Anabolic steroids: Not a good choice—Anabolic steroids are popular forms of synthetic testosterone that have become notorious because of their illicit use—and abuse—by athletes. Anabolic means "having the capacity to build muscle," and this is the reason anabolic steroids were developed—to help seriously ill people rebuild muscle. Anabolic steroids increase the conversion of nitrogen in protein food to muscle. They have legitimate uses as prescription drugs, but they can have harmful side effects, which become worse at higher doses. This often happens with athletes who overdose on steroids or use two or more steroids at the same time. Harmful side effects include a significant risk of heart or liver disease and high blood pressure for both men and women. When taken by women, anabolic steroids can cause masculinizing: growth of facial hair, deepening of the voice, male-pattern baldness, and enlargement of the clitoris. They can also disrupt the menstrual cycle and ovulation.

For men, anabolic steroids may cause an initial increase in libido, but it does not last. After a while the hypothalamus stops stimulating the body's production of testosterone since there is plenty of synthetic testosterone circulating in the blood. As a result, the testicles (which normally produce testosterone) shrink. After that, natural testosterone levels drop, resulting in loss of sexual desire and sometimes impotence. Sperm production is impaired, which can result in permanent sterility.

Psychological effects can be devastating and are sometimes called "'roid rage." Steroid abuse can indeed result in rage, as well as aggressiveness, violence, wide mood swings, and even psychotic symptoms.

*Exercise, Sex, and Winning*

Testosterone levels can be stimulated by exercise, sex, competition and victory. Exercise raises testosterone levels for both men and women and boosts the sex drive for both. This increased sex drive is probably not caused solely by higher testosterone levels, unless testosterone was previously low. Other physical and psychological benefits of exercise enhance sex, too.

Sex raises testosterone levels for both sexes, although the increases are higher for women than for men. One study tested testosterone levels in the saliva of four male–female couples both before and after sexual intercourse and also on nights when they did not have intercourse. For both men and women, their levels of testosterone were higher after intercourse.

Competing *and winning* in almost any social activity seems to raise testosterone levels. Winning is important. If you lose, testosterone levels fall. Dr. James M. Dabbs, Jr., a professor in the Department of Psychology at Georgia State University, proved that testosterone affects behavior and vice versa. He found that testosterone levels rise when individuals meet with success in social encounters. When they meet with failure, their testosterone levels fall. When male tennis players and wrestlers lost a match, their testosterone levels fell. When they won, their testosterone rose and remained up through the next match until they lost. This phenomenon has been confirmed in a number of studies; that is, testosterone rises with victory and falls with defeat.

*Testosterone Supplementation*

Testosterone supplementation may be prescribed by a physician to increase a man's sex drive if lab tests show a deficiency. However, it needs to be emphasized that there are *many* possible causes for a diminished interest in sex. Low testosterone is just one of them. In any case, any kind of supplemental hormone therapy needs to be monitored by a physician, partly because increasing the levels of testosterone can increase the risk of certain types of cancer.

Testosterone supplementation is increasingly being prescribed for older men and for women deficient in testosterone. When it is prescribed for women it is often combined with the female hormones estrogen and progesterone. For many people whose testosterone levels are still in the normal range, DHEA may produce the small amount of testosterone they need to restore vitality and enhance libido.

To find out whether or not you are a candidate for hormone supplementation, ask your physician to test your hormone levels. Request a baseline personalized hormone profile.

## ❧ DHEA

DHEA (dehydroepiandrosterone) is a hormone produced by the adrenal glands that can be converted as needed to other hormones. It is an androgen, and is usually converted to testosterone, although it can also be converted to the female hormones. DHEA appears to have other roles as well. It is thought to enhance the immune system; and its rapid decline in the body (which begins at age twenty-five to thirty) appears to be implicated in the process of aging. As DHEA levels fall, symptoms of aging appear—including reduced libido. Does the presence of DHEA prevent the symptoms of aging? Is aging, and perhaps even death, caused by the rapid decline of DHEA? We don't know yet, but DHEA appears to be a bio-marker. This means that its level in the body is a measure of how far the process of aging has progressed.

During youth DHEA is the most abundant steroid hormone in the body. Somewhere between the ages of 25 to 30, the DHEA level begins to drop at the rate of about 2 percent a year. By the age of 90, an individual's DHEA level is only about 5 percent of what it was at its peak. Just before death, the DHEA level is virtually zero.

Does this mean that taking DHEA supplements will reverse the symptoms of aging, restore youthful vigor, and re-activate a dynamic sex life? In the hopes that the answer is yes, consumers have proved more than willing to give it a try. As a result, DHEA supplements are sold virtually everywhere.

Can DHEA supplementation live up to the extravagant claims being made for it? Is DHEA supplementation safe? What is the story behind DHEA? The public interest in DHEA raises many questions.

## DHEA: Questions and Answers

*Q. Who should consider taking DHEA?*
Usually DHEA supplementation is not advised for younger people unless prescribed by a physician. The labels on DHEA supplements will sometimes say not to use DHEA if you are below the age of forty. Ordinarily, you need not think about taking supplementary DHEA until levels begin to decline naturally with age. Since DHEA can raise levels of testosterone and estrogen, it is not recommended for anyone who has a type of cancer that is hormone dependent (such as prostate cancer or breast cancer).

*Q. What claims are made for DHEA?*
The benefits claimed for DHEA are like those for testosterone and estrogen—DHEA triggers the production of small amounts of testosterone or estrogen, whichever is needed to restore more youthful levels.

DHEA is said to:

- Enhance or revive the sex drive
- Increase energy and motivation
- Elevate mood
- Reduce stress
- Fight fatigue and depression
- Burn fat
- Increase muscle mass
- Help erase fine wrinkles
- Help "dry eye"
- Improve memory
- Strengthen the immune system
- Prevent heart disease

*Q. What evidence supports claims that DHEA enhances sex?*
Evidence is primarily anecdotal from doctors who have prescribed DHEA as well as from DHEA users. Men report that it increases their interest in sex and improves their sexual performance. Some older males who had not had morning erections for years began to experience them again after taking DHEA. Women report increases in libido even more frequently than men do. This might be because DHEA raises testosterone levels in women more than in men, who already have high testosterone levels.

In addition to enhancing the physical aspects of sex, DHEA treats the emotional aspects as well. It promotes feelings of happiness and well-being, fights depression, and replaces it with optimism. All of these positive emotions contribute toward an active, satisfying sex life.

*Q. Will taking DHEA "masculinize" women?*
Clinical trials with women over 40 showed that taking even 50 mg of DHEA per day (the usual dosage for males) raised testosterone levels only to those normal in healthy young women. This is because both testosterone and DHEA levels decline sharply with age. A forty-year-old woman has a testosterone level that is about half that of a twenty-year-old. Very high doses of DHEA, however, can be cause for concern. Researchers found that a 300 mg oral dose of crystalline DHEA will raise testosterone levels high enough to cause masculinizing effects such as growth of facial hair and lowering of the voice. The dosage usually taken by women is up to 25 mg per day.

## ∾ ESTROGEN

Estrogen is usually thought of as the primary female hormone. Actually, estrogen is not just one hormone, but a class of hormones. An estrogen is a hormone that causes estrus (proliferation of cells in the lining of the uterus to prepare for pregnancy). At first, scientists thought there was only one hormone that did this and named it estrogen. Now we know that there are at least three: estrone, estradiol, and estriol. The first two are fairly potent estrogens. Estriol is the weakest.

### Production of Estrogens
Estrogens are produced in the ovaries, the adrenal glands, and in the placenta of a developing fetus. They are also produced by fat and muscle cells, even after menopause, when the ovaries stop producing estrogen. That is why obese women often have high estrogen levels even after menopause. Estrogens (and

hormones in general) are such potent chemicals that the body only needs to secrete minute amounts. In her entire lifetime a woman produces barely two tablespoons of estrogen and progesterone. Like the production of testosterone, the production of the estrogens is ultimately controlled by the hypothalamus in the brain.

### Phytoestrogens and Xenoestrogens

In recent years researchers have discovered chemicals in plants and pollutants in the environment that act like estrogens when they enter our bodies. These are called phytoestrogens (plant estrogens) and xenoestrogens (chemical compounds in the environment that act like estrogens). Finally, there are synthetic and natural estrogens produced by pharmaceutical companies and available by prescription.

#### Phytoestrogens

Phytoestrogens have a mild estrogen action and have been used for menopausal symptoms. Some plant sources of phytoestrogens are tropical wild yams (*Dioscorea*), soybeans, vegetables in the cabbage family, and the herbs dong quai and black cohosh.

#### Xenoestrogens

Xenoestrogens are commonly found in products and byproducts derived from petrochemicals such as fuel oil, heating oil, pesticides, herbicides, plastics, and dioxins—to name just a few out of the thousands. Some of these have extremely potent estrogenic action, powerful enough to be toxic. There is a growing body of research suggesting that they may be implicated in causing breast, ovarian, and testicular cancer, infertility, low sperm count, and feminization of males. Most breast cancer is dependent on estrogen. Thus it does not seem unreasonable to suspect that breast cancer could be triggered or accelerated by environmental pollutants that act like potent estrogens when they enter the body.

This is a powerful reason to clean up the environment—especially of petrochemical byproducts.

## Estrogen: Questions and Answers

*Q. How does estrogen affect female sexual development?*
Estrogen is responsible for development of female sex characteristics, regulating the menstrual cycle, and preparing the uterus for pregnancy.

At the onset of puberty, the hypothalamus in the brain initiates a chain of hormonal messages that result in rising estrogen levels. Estrogen then causes the changes that turn a girl into a woman: a growth spurt, broadening of the pelvis, rounding of the hips, development of the breasts, depositing of fat under the skin (which softens it), and the beginning of menstruation.

*Q. How does estrogen affect a woman's sexual desire and response?*
Estrogen does not seem to have much influence on a woman's sexual desire or response, since removal of the ovaries (which effectively stops estrogen production) does not lessen a woman's sex drive or responsiveness. However, estrogen facilitates the physical aspects of sexual intercourse by maintaining the condition of the vaginal lining, providing vaginal lubrication, and preserving the elasticity of the vagina.

*Q. How does the drop of estrogen at menopause affect sexual desire?*
The rapid decline of hormones associated with menopause can cause a myriad of physical and emotional problems that inhibit sex. The drop in estrogen reduces the supply of blood to the vagina and its surrounding tissues. This causes the vaginal lining to become thinner and drier, less able to produce lubricating secretions before and during intercourse. Cracks and lacerations can appear in the vaginal walls. Vaginal infections such as trichomonal vaginitis and pelvic diseases

increase with the loss of estrogen. The vagina shrinks. It loses elasticity and tone, making sex less enjoyable for both the woman and her partner. Gradually the genital tissues lose fat and moisture, flattening out. These tissue changes, along with low hormone levels, are thought to be physically linked to a decline in sexual desire. The breasts change texture and decrease in size. Bladder problems arise, causing fear of incontinence. Muscle mass is lost and fat deposits increase, especially on the hips. Hot flashes occur unpredictably, causing discomfort and sometimes profuse sweating.

In addition to these physical problems, the loss of hormones can bring emotional distress—insomnia, anxiety, irritability, mood swings, depression. The congruence of all these symptoms—physical and emotional—explains why estrogen is the most widely prescribed drug in the United States. Some ten million American women are taking it.

*Q. What about estrogen replacement therapy?*
Estrogen replacement therapy, or ERT, is increasingly being prescribed to relieve the symptoms of menopause, prevent osteoporosis, and protect against heart disease. With ERT, women who have found sexual intercourse uncomfortable because of vaginal drying and changes caused by menopause are once again able to enjoy sex. But ERT has other positive benefits for sex, as well, including relief of the emotional symptoms of menopause. It does not take long for ERT to take effect. Symptoms not only disappear but are reversed within several weeks.

In 1998 a new kind of synthetic estrogen became available for ERT, a so-called "smart estrogen" or "designer estrogen." It has the advantages of estrogen without increasing the risk for uterine or breast cancer or causing monthly uterine bleeding. It may even help prevent breast cancer. Like the body's own estrogen, smart estrogen helps build denser bones and lowers cholesterol. It does not, however, relieve hot flashes, and it appears to be somewhat less effective than regular estrogen supplements in improving bone density and cholesterol. Raloxifene, manufactured by Eli Lilly, was the first smart estrogen approved for marketing in the United States.

ERT usually includes supplemental progesterone (progestins) to counteract the risk of uterine cancer. Sometimes small amounts of testosterone are also used, depending on individual hormone levels. Even though estrogen does not have a direct effect on the sex drive, progesterone and testosterone do. Consequently, the mix of sex hormones included in hormone replacement therapy (HRT) often produces very positive results for a woman's sex life.

DHEA supplementation remains another option for women in menopause, since DHEA can trigger the production of a small amount of estrogen, if needed.

Risks as well as benefits are involved in hormonal supplementation. These need to be discussed with your physician or other health care provider.

Today there are options to traditional ERT: natural hormones, plant estrogens, and herbal alternatives. These are discussed in the interview with Dr. Merey that concludes this chapter.

*Q. Do men produce estrogen?*
Men produce some estrogen, but their estrogen levels are much lower than those of women, while their testosterone levels are much higher. Strangely enough, older men produce more estrogen than postmenopausal women do. Estrogen is thought to help protect against Alzheimer's disease. Since elderly women are three times more likely than men to develop Alzheimer's, some researchers believe that this higher estrogen level in older men may be the reason.

*Q. Do men ever need estrogen supplementation?*
Men do produce some estrogen and progesterone, just as women produce testosterone. Men's levels of those female hormones do not decline with age, however, and do not need to be supplemented.

## ❧ PROGESTERONE

Progesterone and the estrogens comprise the female hormones. Though there are three kinds of estrogen, there is only one progesterone. Its name is derived from *pro* and *gesterone*, meaning "for gestation." Progesterone is produced in huge amounts by the placenta during gestation (pregnancy). It is also produced in the adrenal glands and in the corpus luteum. (The corpus luteum is a cluster of cells left in the ovary after an egg is expelled. This cluster of cells secretes hormones and then degenerates if a pregnancy does not occur.)

## *Progesterone: Questions and Answers*

*Q. How does progesterone affect a woman's sexuality?*
Progesterone works with estrogen and enhances its effects. Unlike estrogen, it seems to affect a woman's sexual desire. It certainly affects her emotions, making her feel good, and hence "sexier." Natural progesterone is a mild tranquilizer, a mood-elevator, and a natural antidepressant that promotes a woman's feeling of well-being. In high enough doses, it is an anesthetic. (Synthetic progesterone, or progestins, on the other hand, can have the opposite effect.) Natural progesterone is available by prescription, as are the progestins.

*Q. Does progesterone, like other sex hormones, decline with age?*
Yes. By the time a woman reaches her thirties, her progesterone levels begin to decline. She may have erratic menstrual cycles and some cycles in which ovulation does not occur. Thus there is no ruptured egg cell to produce progesterone and no monthly surge in progesterone levels. These abnormal cycles become more frequent as menopause approaches. After menopause, when ovulation stops, progesterone production is virtually nil.

*Q. What is the difference between "natural" and "synthetic" progesterone?*

"Natural progesterone" is not made by nature as its name implies, but is produced in a laboratory. It is identical in chemical structure to the hormone produced by the human body. Natural progesterone is available over the counter in cream form containing less than 3 percent progesterone.

Synthetic progesterones are not chemically identical to progesterone produced by the human body. However, they act like progesterone in the body, and, like human progesterone, help protect against uterine cancer. Synthetic progesterones are called progestins. The brand most often prescribed in the United States is Provera.

Progestins are synthesized from a compound found in wild yams. At one time progestin was considered superior to natural progesterone because the form of natural progesterone then available was not as readily absorbed by the body. This is no longer the case. Today's natural progesterone undergoes a process called micronization, which breaks it up into tiny particles that are easily absorbed. Micronized progesterone is now used in all oral preparations, such as capsules.

## ❧ OPTIONS FOR ENHANCING THE SEX DRIVE AFTER MENOPAUSE OR HORMONAL DECLINE: AN INTERVIEW WITH DAISY MEREY, MD, PHD

During mid-life, declining hormone levels can be a great source of sexual problems. Menopause causes a drastic hormonal decline in women. Hormonal decline is much less dramatic in men, but can still result in decreased sexual desire. In the following interview, which I conducted with Dr. Merey in 1997, she discusses some of the options available, including traditional and natural hormonal replacement therapy for women and hormone supplementation for men.

Dr. Merey wears many hats. She is a practicing bariatric physician (the medical specialty of weight loss), a Diplomate of the American Society of Bariatric Physicians (one of sixty-five in the United States), and Past International President of the International Academy of Bariatric Physicians. In addition, she is a Fellow of the American Academy of Family Physician and a member of its Cancer Board, President of the Female Physicians of Palm Beach County, Florida, and on that organization's committee for Women's Health Issues. In addition, she is an Associate Bionutrition Consultant who lectures frequently on the choices available for hormonal replacement therapy and on the connections between neurotransmitters and weight control. Her practice is located in West Palm Beach, Florida.

*Q. Dr. Merey, how do you feel about hormone replacement therapy?*
*Merey:* Well, it all depends on each person's needs. Everyone is an individual. But after the age of forty, all our hormones start decreasing—estrogen, progesterone, and testosterone. Females have a larger preponderance of estrogen and progesterone, and males of testosterone, but as we get older, unfortunately, all those levels decline.

*Q. What are some of the symptoms of a low hormone level in women?*
*Merey*: There are a number of symptoms: depression, insomnia, hot flashes, difficulty concentrating, dizziness. Sometimes husbands will report that their wives are very irritable, jumping on them for every little thing. Often when we test the patient's hormone level we find that the hormones are out of balance. Some women need estrogen; some need progesterone; some need only DHEA (an androgen); some need a combination of all three. Some women's bodies produce all the hormones they need from the adrenal glands, body fat, and so on, and don't require hormone replacement at all.

Another symptom of a hormonal problem is lack of sexual desire, which can indicate low testosterone. Testosterone increases libido—for women also, not just for men. Thus testosterone can be added to a woman's hormonal regime.

*Q. What about men? What would lead you to suspect that a man's testosterone level is low?*

*Merey:* We check testosterone level in a man's blood when he complains of lack of libido. When a man says that all his life his libido has been fine and then suddenly it is not, there are two probable reasons. He may not be attracted to his partner. Or, his hormone levels may be decreasing. Thus the first thing we do when a man has a loss of libido is check his hormone levels. If we find that his testosterone level is low, we try to supplement it.

There is also the problem of impotence. But that is a bit more complicated than lack of libido. With impotence, men may have the desire to have sexual intercourse, but have a mechanical problem, which cannot be treated hormonally.

*Q. What about the risk of prostate cancer? Would you have to do a PSA test before you prescribe testosterone or DHEA?*

*Merey:* We definitely would not give testosterone to a patient who has prostate cancer because testosterone stimulates prostate cancer. DHEA supplementation is a bit controversial. Some investigators think you can't give it to patients who have prostate cancer. Others think you can. Some say that DHEA even improves the state of the patient who has prostate cancer. Others say you shouldn't use it at all. I would use it with caution, because DHEA gives patients a feeling of well-being. But I would continue checking it, monitoring the patient, because DHEA is a hormone precursor. It is a precursor of estrogen, progesterone, and testosterone—a precursor of all sex hormones.

*Q. What tests should a woman have before you would prescribe supplemental hormones?*

*Merey:* Women need a mammogram and a Pap smear just to rule out the risk of cancer before starting hormone replacement therapy—or even DHEA supplementation.

*Q. Is it possible to overdose on DHEA? Should you have your DHEA level tested before you take it?*

*Merey:* I definitely prefer for the patient to have the DHEA level tested because we have had a large array of DHEA levels in patients. Some patients have had very low levels of DHEA; others have had high levels. People who have a high level of DHEA in their blood should not be taking more.

*Q. Is that true even for older people?*

*Merey:* We have had older people who have had a high DHEA level in their blood. In general, I feel that women may take 25 mg of DHEA daily. Men may take up to 50 mg. But before going to 50 mg they should consult a physician who can monitor that amount.

*Q. What are your thoughts about estrogen and progesterone supplementation—the pros and the cons?*

*Merey:* Estrogen is good for bone density and it improves cardiovascular activity. It is good for the skin; it helps the hair. It increases longevity not only for women, but for men. Men who are on estrogen also live longer. On the other hand, with estrogen you have the risk of cancer—cancer of the uterus. That's why you have to balance estrogen with progesterone.

Progesterone is very good for preventing cancer of the endometrium (lining of the uterus). If you give women estrogen, you have to balance it with progesterone. The problem is that progesterone can cause cancer of the breast. So you are walking on a tightrope. You don't want women to have cancer of the uterus; you don't want them to have cancer of the breast.

If women don't have a uterus because of a hysterectomy, you don't have to give them progesterone to protect against uterine cancer. Progesterone helps prevent uterine cancer but can increase the risk for breast cancer.

The risk for cancer of the breast from hormone replacement therapy is 1 percent, but that is still high if you happen to be in that 1 percent! Researchers have found that more women die from fractures—especially hip fractures—than from breast cancer. Estrogen protects against osteoporosis, which causes bone loss and fractures. The mortality rate for women who *don't* take estrogen is higher than for women who do. Thus scientists feel that hormone replacement therapy saves lives.

*Q. I have seen estrogen creams for sale in health food stores. How do you feel about trying an over-the-counter estrogen product to see if it relieves, say, menopausal symptoms?*
*Merey:* Well, I don't think it's detrimental if you use a *phyto-estrogen*, like the estrogen in dong quai or black cohosh, which are both herbs. Those are not detrimental. They are phyto-estrogens—estrogens from plant sources. The extract of black cohosh, for example, has been extensively studied in Germany. It is used for relief of perimenopausal depression, vaginal dryness, and mood swings. It is a safe, nonhormonal way for women with a family history of breast, uterine, or ovarian cancer to get relief from perimenopausal symptoms. [Perimenopause is the transitional period of approximately two to five years preceding menopause.]

*Q. Have you had patients that actually improved by taking black cohosh?*
*Merey:* Absolutely. We've had even *husbands* thanking us. Black cohosh has been used in Germany for fifty years. So it is not something new.

*Q. What other natural products do you like?*
*Merey:* I like estriol, which is a very mild form of estrogen with wild yam extract. Estriol cream is a natural estrogen product with an excellent local effect. When it is applied to the genital area, it can relieve vaginal dryness and painful intercourse without the risk of breast, uterine, or ovarian cancer. The cream is absorbed through the skin, but because it does not

combine with nuclear estrogen receptors in the body's cells, it doesn't act as a growth factor [for cancer].

*Q. Is it true that Asian women who eat a lot of soy products don't have as many menopausal symptoms?*
*Merey:* That is correct. The soy supplement also stimulates bone mass density, relieves hot flashes, and prevents cancer in both men and women—not only cancer of the breast and uterus but also cancer of the prostate. There is a new study in which scientists are feeding soy products to men to prevent cancer of the prostate.

*Q. Soy is not really an estrogen then, but it prevents symptoms of menopause?*
*Merey:* The soy product is a phytohormone. *Phyto* means "plant." What it does is stimulate bone density and prevent cancer—cancer of the breast and of the uterus and of the prostate. We have found that there are a lot of phytohormones that have the *good*, the advantageous side effects of the hormone, and not the negative side effects—one of which is the production of cancer, which is unfortunately what happens with estrogen.

*Q. So this is why you like to prescribe phytoestrogens?*
*Merey:* We try to do as much as possible with natural estrogen. We feel that definitely we don't want women to have any problems with their bones, because apparently three times as many women die from hip fractures as from cancer of the breast or the uterus.

On the other hand, you have to be very careful and monitor the patients. You have to have them get mammograms and Pap smears and make sure everything is okay. Once you start a patient on hormone replacement therapy, you must continue checking her.

However, a new medication is available, a "smart estrogen." Smart estrogens are estrogen-like products that stimulate all the good side effects of estrogen, but they are not cancer producing.

Now that there will be more postmenopausal women in the population, it definitely behooves drug companies to do more studies on hormone replacement therapy.

In general, we feel that women often need hormone replacement therapy. The main thing to emphasize is that there are many options available. A lot of women don't know that there is anything else but Premarin, which is a widely prescribed cross-species estrogen from horses. Premarin is a mixture of over twenty different estrogens taken from the urine of pregnant mares.

There is evidence to suggest that the byproducts of the metabolic breakdown of Premarin (called "daughter compounds") are stronger than the equine estrogens themselves. When you use a hormone that is native to the female body, such as estradiol, the body will metabolize it into weaker "daughter" compounds—but with Premarin the daughter compounds get stronger and have the potential to cause more side effects. We really don't know the effects of this—especially high doses—over a long period of time. Then too, with Premarin there is the controversial issue of how the mares are cared for on the farms that collect their urine.

But there are a lot of options available. You don't *have* to take Premarin or a similar compound. If you have cancer in your family and you don't want to take synthetic estrogen, you can take other things. There are phytoestrogens. There are natural hormones. There are herbal alternatives. All women can weigh what they want to do. The best thing to do is to discuss it with somebody you trust. I am sure there are many physicians who have the same program as I do. There are a lot of supplements available and things are constantly changing. I think it's because drug companies realize that we women live longer now and that we need medications to keep us healthy.

*Q. What about progesterone? Are there natural alternatives to synthetic progesterones such as Provera?*

*Merey:* Yes, there is natural progesterone. Natural progesterone still protects your uterus and breasts from the effects of excess estrogen but has no side effects when taken in appropriate doses. And it does not adversely affect your blood triglycerides and cholesterol. Natural progesterone helps build strong bones and has a calming effect on the central nervous system. Better yet, it is a precursor hormone that your body can use to create other hormones.

If you are currently on Provera—a synthetic form of progesterone—chances are good that you have been given this to protect your uterus from excess buildup of tissue from estrogen. Provera does a good job of protecting the endometrial lining in this way, but it is not the same as natural progesterone—which is often a better choice. Provera can cause PMS-like symptoms such as weight gain, bloating, headache, and depression.

Many women get relief from hot flashes with a topical natural progesterone cream made from the extract of the wild Mexican yam, such as Pro-Gest cream. It is not known to aggravate estrogen-dependent breast, uterine, or ovarian cancers. Natural progesterone is also available as sublingual, vaginal, or rectal suppositories, and tablets of micronized oil.

*Q. There are so many options available. How can you find out what's right for you?*
*Merey:* Whether you are trying to make a decision about initiating hormone therapy or staying on your current regimen, you'll want to know what your hormone profile looks like. The first step is to get a baseline personalized hormone profile.

Remember, hormone levels should be *physiologic*—not too high, not too low. That is the range your body will feel best with in most circumstances.

Have your doctor order a hormone profile. Then work with your doctor to develop a program that is right for you.

CHAPTER NINE

*Products That Inhibit Sex or*
*Are Worthless as Aphrodisiacs*

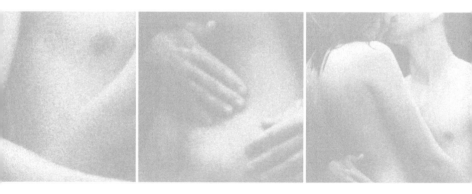

*P*eople often experiment with prescription drugs, mood-altering or hallucinogenic drugs, alcohol, tobacco, or other worthless products marketed as "aphrodisiacs" to enhance their libido. Instead of increasing people's sex drives, these substances inhibit performance and can cause negative and even harmful effects.

## ❧ PRESCRIPTION DRUGS

In addition to over-the-counter barbiturates and amphetamines (found in many diet pills), certain prescription drugs adversely affect sex drive and performance. Classes of prescription drugs that can cause a lowered sex drive or impotence include immunosuppressive agents, antihypertensives, antidepressants, tranquilizers, muscle relaxants, ulcer drugs, and oral contraceptives.

The drugs listed below may cause impotence, according to the American Urological Association. The drug's generic name is listed first, followed by examples of brand names in parentheses. If you are taking any of these drugs, consult your physician to see if an alternate drug could be prescribed.

*Immunosuppressive Agents*
Indomethacin (Indocin), methysergide (Sansert), metoclopramide (Reglan), metronidazole (Flagyl), phenytoin, (Dilantin), procarbazine (Matulane).

*Blood Pressure Medicines and Diuretics*
Thiazides (Diuril, Esidrix, Hygroton), spironolactone (Aldatone), methyldopa (Aldomet), clonidine (Catapres), reserpine (Seracil), guanethidine (Ismelin), pargylin (Eutonyl), phenoxybenzamine (Dibenzaline), phentolamine (Regitine), propanolol (Inderal), metoprolol (Lopressor).

*Anti-anxiety Medications*
Chlordiazepoxide (Librium), oxazepam (Serax), clorazepate (Tranxen), meprobamate (Miltown, Equanil), tybamate (Tybatran).

*Antidepressants*
Nortripotyline (Aventyl), amitriptyline (Elavil), desipramine (Norpramin), doxepin (Sinequan), fluorexetine (Prozac), imipramine (Tofranil, Norfanil, Tipramine), isocargoxazid (Marplan), paroxetine (Paxil), phenelzine (Nardill), sertraline (Zoloft), tranylcypromine (Parnate).

*Tranquilizers*
Diazepam (Valium), fluphenazine (Prolixin), trifluoperazine (Stelazine), prochlorperazine (Compazine), mesoridaxine (Serentil), promazine (Sparine), Chlorpromazine (Thorazine), thiothixene (Navane), chlorprothixine (Taractan).

*Drugs for Bladder or Bowel Spasms*
Proantheline bromide (Pro-Banthine), atropine (usually used in combination with other drugs).

*Drugs for Parkinson's Disease*
Biperidin (Akineton), cycrimine (Pagitane), procyclidine (Kemadrin), trihexyphenidyl (Artane), benztropine (Cogentin), levodopa (Larodopa, Sinemet).

*Drugs for Allergies/Motion Sickness*
Dimenhydrinate (Dramamine), hydroxyzine (Vistaril), meclizine (Antivert, Bonine), promethazine (Phenergan).

*Antifungal Drug*
Ketoconazole (Nizoral).

## ❧ STREET DRUGS, ALCOHOL, AND TOBACCO

Not surprisingly, substances that abuse the body also have an adverse effect on sexual desire and performance. Amphetamines, alcohol, recreational and hard drugs, nicotine, and caffeine have all been used to increase sexual pleasure and desire. In the long run, many of them have the reverse effect.

## Mood-Altering or Hallucinogenic Drugs

The sexual effects of mood-altering drugs such as marijuana, LSD, and cocaine are unpredictable and seem to depend largely on the user's expectations for the drug's effects. While some users claim they enhance sex, they can also magnify negative emotions and preexisting sexual disorders. But while the aphrodisiac powers of these drugs is a matter of debate, their harmful effects on the body are not. (The harmful effects of marijuana are discussed on p. 53.)

### LSD (lysergic acid diethylamide)

LSD is a strong hallucinogen that produces unpredictable emotional experiences—ranging from pleasant to terrifying. Reports on its aphrodisiac powers are also conflicting, but are mostly negative. Since it is an illegal substance, supplies may be "cut" with toxic substances.

### Cocaine

Cocaine is an anesthetic that is used as an aphrodisiac because it stimulates the areas of the brain that control sexual arousal. Although low dosages heighten sexual response, higher dosages inhibit sex by creating fear, paranoia, and aggression. In addition, sexual satisfaction is, at best, long delayed.

Cocaine is highly addictive, and its pleasurable effects cannot be sustained at their initial levels. The body moderates such effects with prolonged usage. Since it is an illegal drug, most supplies are impure. Its dangers far outweigh any positive benefits.

### MDMA (methylenedioxymethamphetamine)

MDMA is also called "ecstasy." It is related to amphetamines and is a mood-enhancer, or "happy pill." Because it releases emotional inhibitions it is used as an aphrodisiac. The problem is that MDMA was withdrawn from medical use in the 1980s. Consequently any supplies are manufactured illegally and may be impure or toxic, and its use is now illegal.

### Volatile Nitrites

For some individuals, a group of chemicals, the volatile nitrites, are said to enhance sexual response and prolong orgasm. These chemicals are absorbed quickly by inhaling. This causes a rush of blood to the brain, which induces sexual stimulation but can also cause fatal cerebral hemorrhage. These chemicals are sometimes marketed as "room deodorizers." (Even for this purported use they are not safe, since they are highly flammable.)

### Amyl Nitrite

Amyl nitrite is also known as "poppers." It dilates the blood vessels and is used as an inhalant to treat angina. Its reputation as an aphrodisiac comes from its use by homosexuals to prolong orgasm and relax the anal sphincter muscle.

Amyl nitrite causes the heart to race wildly and blood pressure to drop dramatically, even in healthy individuals. Amyl nitrate can also inhibit the immune system.

## Alcohol

Alcohol is commonly thought of an aphrodisiac, partly because it can release inhibitions. But alcohol has its down side. Even moderate amounts of alcohol can impair a man's ability to sustain an erection. Excessive amounts over a period of time can lower levels of the male sex hormone testosterone, depress sexual reflexes, and cause sexual dysfunction. It can also damage the liver, which raises estrogen levels and can cause impotence. As Shakespeare says of alcohol in *Macbeth*: "It provokes the desire, but it takes away the performance." However, a small amount of alcohol can help release inhibitions or anxiety connected with sex. The British are fond of downing a shot of gin spiked with pepper to spice up their love life.

## Tobacco

Smoking or chewing tobacco decreases sexual function in men because the nicotine it contains constricts blood vessels. Not only does it harm the entire cardiovascular system, but specifically, nicotine reduces blood flow into the penis. According to Irving J. Fishman, MD, associate professor of urology at Baylor University School of Medicine, smoking just two cigarettes a day can inhibit an erection. He says "If you measure the blood flow in a man's penis and then have him smoke a cigarette, you'll see a dramatic fall."

The Centers for Disease Control and Prevention conducted a study of 4,400 men, which showed that smokers had a rate of impotence at least 50 percent higher than men who did not smoke. This was true even after considering all other risk factors for impotence, such as depression, anxiety, age, and alcoholism. According to the study, the risk of smoking-caused impotence increased with age. The critical ages are between thirty and fifty.

The good news is that erectile function is substantially improved once men stop smoking. Dr. Alexander Olshanyetsky of the Jerusalem Impotency and Fertility Medical Center said that of his patients who took his advice and quit smoking, approximately 80 percent reported improvement in their ability to attain an erection. This occurred two to six months after they quit smoking. After a year of not smoking and avoiding tobacco smoke, 90 percent reported almost normal sexual function.

Another sexually squelching effect of smoking is that the smell might turn off a non-smoking partner. One study of non-smokers determined that 80 percent of women and 65 percent of men are turned off sexually by the odor of a partner who smokes. Of the 5,500 non-smoking women surveyed, 45 percent said they definitely would not have sex with a partner who smokes; 25 percent said they would have sex with smokers, but that they would have sex more often and enjoy it more if their partners did not smoke.

# ❧ WORTHLESS PRODUCTS MARKETED AS "APHRODISIACS"

Since January 6, 1990, the FDA has banned interstate commerce and over-the-counter (OTC) sales of any products that claim on their label to arouse or increase sexual desire or improve sexual performance. The FDA's position is that "there is a lack of adequate data to establish general recognition of the safety and effectiveness of any of these ingredients, or any other ingredient, for OTC use as an aphrodisiac. Labeling claims for OTC use as aphrodisiacs are either false, misleading, or unsupported by scientific data."

The FDA ban does not extend to products such as ginseng, which are generally thought to be aphrodisiacs but are not promoted as such. In spite of the ban, there are countless formulas, substances, and devices advertised to rejuvenate sexual potency or cure impotence. The United States Postal Service can seize them under Title 39, U.S. Code 30005, on a charge of false representation in promoting a scheme or device to obtain money or property through the mail. But it is easy to change a company's or product's name and sell the product again. New "miracle cures" pop up every day in the classified ads of the tabloids. Consumer beware!

Examples of worthless aphrodisiacs seized by the Postal Service include:

- Big Ox
- European Love Drops
- Instant Love Potion
- Linga Pendulum Penis Enlarger and Strengthener
- Mad Dog Weed
- Mexican Spanish Fly in Liquid Form
- Super Nature Tablets

# Afterword

One final word. Practice safe sex. Nothing can be more inhibiting to enjoyable sex or turn off a partner more quickly than having to worry about the possible consequences of sex—whether it be a sexually transmitted disease or an unwanted pregnancy.

# Resource List

**Laboratories**

The following laboratories do saliva testing for DHEA:

Aeron Life Cycles
1933 Davis St.
San Leandro, CA 94566
Phone: 1-800-631-7900 or 510-729-0375

Diagnos-Techs, Inc.
6620 S. 192nd Place, Suite J-104
Kent, WA 98032
Phone: 1-800-878-3787 or 425-251-0596

**Health Practitioners and Associations**

American Holistic Medical Association
67628 Old McClean Village Drive
McClean, VA 22101
Phone: 919-787-5146

American Urological Association, Inc.
1120 North Charles Street
Baltimore, MD 21201
Phone: 410-727-1100

The Herb Research Foundation
1007 Pearl Street, Suite 200
Boulder, CO 80302
Phone: 303-449-2265
Fax: 303-449-7849
E-mail: info@herbs.org

National Association for Holistic Aromatherapy
P.O. Box 17622
Boulder, CO 80308
Phone: 888-ASK-NAHA
Phone: 314-963-2071
Fax: 314-963-4454
http://www.naha.org
Email: info@naha.org

Dr. Daisy Merey, MD, PhD
200 Butler Street, Suite 201
West Palm Beach, FL 33401
Phone: (561) 659-6756

## Further Reading

### *Aromatherapy and Fragrance*

Damian, Peter and Kate. *Aromatherapy: Scent and Psyche.* Rochester, VT: Healing Arts Press, 1995.

Davis, Patricia. *Aromatherapy: An A–Z.* Essex, England: C. W. Daniel Co., Ltd., 1988.

Keville, Kathi. *Pocket Guide to Aromatherapy.* Freedom, CA: The Crossing Press, 1993.

Keville, Kathi and Mindy Green. *Aromatherapy: A Complete Guide to the Healing Art.* Freedom, CA: The Crossing Press, 1995.

Lacroix, Nitya with Sakina Bowhay. *The Art of Sensual Aromatherapy: A Lover's Guide to Using Aromatic Oils and Essences.* New York: Henry Holt, 1995.

Lawless, Julia. *The Encyclopedia of Essential Oils: The Complete Guide to the Use of Aromatics in Aromatherapy, Herbalism, Health & Well-Being.* Rockport, MA: Element Books, Inc., 1992.

Moran, Jan. *Fabulous Fragrances: How to Select Your Perfume Wardrobe—The Woman's Guide to Prestige Perfumes.*

Beverly Hills, CA: Crescent House, 1994.

Rose, Jeanne. *The Aromatherapy Book: Applications & Inhalations.* Berkeley, CA: North Atlantic Books, 1992.

Wildwood, Christine. *The Aromatherapy and Massage Book.* London, England: Thorson, an imprint of HarperCollins, 1993.

Worwood, Valerie Ann. *The Fragrant Mind: Aromatherapy for Personality, Mind, Mood, and Emotion.* Novato, CA: New World Library, 1996.

### Herbs

Crawford, Amanda McQuade. *The Herbal Menopause Book: Herbs, Nutrition, and Other Natural Remedies.* Freedom, CA: The Crossing Press, 1996.

Green, James. *The Male Herbal: Health Care for Men & Boys.* Freedom, CA: The Crossing Press, 1991.

Hoffman, David. *The Information Sourcebook of Herbal Medicine.* Freedom, CA: The Crossing Press, 1994.

Hopman, Ellen Evert. *A Druid's Herbal for the Sacred Earth Year.* Rochester, NY: Destiny Books, 1995.

Mayell, Mark. *Off-the-Shelf Natural Health: How to Use Herbs and Nutrients to Stay Well.* NY: Bantam Books, 1995.

Meyer, Clarence. *Herbal Aphrodisiacs from World Sources.* Glenwood, IL: Meyerbooks, 1993.

Rose, Jeanne. *Herbs & Aromatherapy for the Reproductive System.* Berkeley, CA: Frog, Ltd., 1994.

Ryman, Danièle. *The Aromatherapy Handbook: The Secret Healing Power of Essential Oils.* Essex, England: C. W. Daniel Company Ltd., 1984.

St. Claire, Debra. *Pocket Herbal Reference Guide.* Freedom, CA: The Crossing Press, 1993.

Santillo, Humbart. *Natural Healing with Herbs.* Prescott, AZ: Hohm Press, 1984.

Tierra, Lesley. *Healing with Chinese Herbs*. Freedom, CA: The Crossing Press, 1997.

Tierra, Lesley. *The Herbs of Life: Health and Healing Using Western & Chinese Techniques*. Freedom, CA: The Crossing Press, 1992.

### Human Sexuality

Kelly, Gary F. *Sexuality Today: The Human Perspective*, Fifth Edition. NY: McGraw Hill, 1995.

Masters, William H., Virginia E. Johnson, and Robert C. Kolodny. *Human Sexuality*, Fourth Edition. NY: HarperCollins, 1992.

Reinisch, June M. and Ruth Beasley. *The Kinsey Institute New Report on Sex*. NY: St. Martin's Press, 1990.

### Neurotransmitters and Hormones

Cherniske, Stephen. *The DHEA Breakthrough*. NY: Ballantine Books, 1996.

Rako, Susan. *The Hormone of Desire: The Truth About Sexuality, Menopause, and Testosterone*. NY: Harmony Books, 1996.

Regelson, William and Carol Colman. *The Super-Hormone Promise: Nature's Antidote to Aging*. NY: Simon & Schuster, 1996.

Winter, Ruth. *The Anti-Aging Hormones That Can Help You Beat the Clock*. NY: Three Rivers Press, 1997.

### Nutrition

Balch, James E. and Phyllis A. Balch. *Prescription for Nutritional Healing*. NY: Avery Publishing Group, 1990.

Carper, Jean. *Food—Your Miracle Medicine: How Food Can Prevent and Cure Over 100 Symptoms and Problems*. NY: HarperCollins, 1993.

Cooper, Kenneth H. *Advanced Nutritional Therapies.* Nashville: Thomas Nelson, 1996.

Davis, Adelle. *Let's Get Well.* NY: The Penguin Group, 1965.

Dunne, Lavon J. *Nutrition Almanac.* NY: McGraw Hill, 1990.

Mayell, Mark. *Off-the-Shelf Natural Health: How to Use Herbs and Nutrients to Stay Well.* NY: Bantam Books, 1995.

Prevention Magazine, eds. *The Complete Book of Vitamins and Minerals for Health.* Emmaus, PA: Rodale Press, 1988.

Quillin, Patrick. *Healing Nutrients.* Chicago: Contemporary Books, 1987.

Reader's Digest, eds. *Foods That Harm: Foods That Heal.* Pleasantville, NY: The Reader's Digest Association, 1997.

Walker, Morton. *Sexual Nutrition.* Garden City Park, NY: Avery Publishing, 1994.

### Pheromones

Kohl, James Vaughn and Robert T. Francoeur. *The Scent of Eros: Mysteries of Odor in Human Sexuality.* NY: Continuum, 1995.

### General Works

Crenshaw, Theresa L. *The Alchemy of Love and Lust.* NY: G. P. Putnam's Sons, 1996.

Lamm, Steven. *Younger at Last: The New World of Vitality Medicine.* NY: Simon & Schuster, 1997.

Mayell, Mark. *Off-the-Shelf Natural Health: How to Use Herbs and Nutrients to Stay Well.* NY: Bantam Books, 1995.

Page, Linda Rector. *Healthy Healing*, Tenth Edition. Carmel Valley, CA: Healthy Healing Publications, 1997.

Pearson, Durk and Sandy Shaw. *Life Extension: A Practical Scientific Approach.* NY: Warner Books, Inc., 1982.

Pitchford, Paul. *Healing with Whole Foods: Oriental Traditions and Modern Nutrition*, Revised Edition. Berkeley, CA: North Atlantic Books, 1993.

Watson, Cyntha Mervis, MD, with Angela Hynes. *Love Potions*. New York: G.P. Putnam's Sons, 1993.

Weill, Andrew. *8 Weeks to Optimum Health*. NY: Alfred A. Knopf, 1997.

Werthheimer, Neil, ed. *Total Health for Men*. Emmaus, PA: Rodale Press, 1995.

# Index

nutrients
as aphrodisiacs, 16, 87-98
boosting hormone levels
with, 138, 144-146
boosting neurotransmitter
levels with, 112-114,
121-122, 125-126
taken prior to lovemaking,
87-94
taken regularly for sexual
vigor, 94-98
nux vomica, 11

## O
oats, 42
omega-3 fatty acids, 97
orgasm, stage of sexual
response, 15, 16
oxytocin, 135

## P
pantothenic acid, 99
patchouli, 39
pepper, 82
peptides, 134, 135
perfume, 61, 66
phenylalanine, 91-92, 112, 115,
124
phenylethylamine (PEA), 93-94
pheromones, 135-136
as aphrodisiacs, 57-67
discovery of human, 58
female, 60, 63
human production of, 60
in male and female scents,
60, 65, 66
in smellprints, 61, 66

male, 60, 62-63
using to enhance sex, 61,
64
phytoestrogens, 151, 160, 161,
162
phytohormones, 161
pills, herbal, 47
poison nut, 54
positive thinking, 129, 139
Premarin, 162
progesterone,134, 136, 154,
155-156, 157, 158, 159
prostaglandins, 97
prostate, 23
protein, 95, 112-113
Provera, 156, 163
Prozac, 119, 120, 123
pyridoxine, 100

## R
REM sleep, 17
response, stages of sexual, 15-18
riboflavin, 99
rose, 79-81

## S
sandalwood, 81
sanguinaria, 11
sarsaparilla, 43
saw palmetto, 23, 43
scents
erotic, 63, 73-81
mood-enhancing, 82, 83
soothing, 61, 83
stimulating to senses, 61,
82
schisandra, 44

# RELATED BOOKS BY THE CROSSING PRESS

## 200 Ways to Love the Body You Have
By Marcia Hutchinson

This companion to Marcia Hutchinson's *Transforming Body Image* consists of 200 pleasurable exercises from which you can choose at random. The exercises encourage you to become focused and aware of your body as it is, leading you to love the body you have.

$12.95 • Paper • ISBN 0-89594-999-7

## Aromatherapy: *A Complete Guide to the Healing Art*
By Kathi Keville and Mindy Green

This complete guide presents everything you need to know to enhance your health, beauty, and emotional well-being through the practice of aromatherapy. Kathi Keville and Mindy Green offer a fresh perspective on the most fragrant of the healing arts.

$16.95 • Paper • ISBN 0-89594-692-0

## Chakras and Their Archetypes: *Uniting Energy Awareness and Spiritual Growth*
By Ambika Wauters

Linking classic archetypes to the seven chakras in the human energy system can reveal unconscious ways of behaving. Wauters helps us understand where our energy is blocked, which attitudes or emotional issues are responsible, and how to then transcend our limitations.

$16.95 • Paper • ISBN 0-89594-891-5

## Clear Mind, Open Heart: *Healing Yourself, Your Relationships and the Planet*
By Eddie and Debbie Shapiro

The Shapiros offer an uplifting, inspiring, and deeply sensitive approach to healing through spiritual awareness. Includes practical exercises and techniques to help us all in making our own journey.

$16.95 • Paper • ISBN 0-89594-917-2

## Essential Reiki: *A Complete Guide to an Ancient Healing Art*
By Diane Stein

This bestseller includes the history of Reiki, hand positions, giving treatments, and the initiations. While no book can replace directly received attunements, Essential Reiki provides everything else that the practitioner and teacher of this system needs, including all three degrees of Reiki, most of it in print for the first time.

$18.95 • Paper • ISBN 0-89594-736-6

# RELATED BOOKS BY THE CROSSING PRESS

## Handbook of Natural Therapies: *Exploring the Spiral of Healing*

By Marcia Starck

When we are troubled by an ailment not suited to treatment by allopathic or conventional Western medicine, what can we do? In this book, Starck discusses nearly fifty therapies that can be used in a holistic approach to health.

$14.95 • Paper • ISBN 0-89594-869-9

## The Healing Energy of Your Hands

By Michael Bradford

Bradford offers techniques so simple that anyone can work with healing energy quickly and easily.

$12.95 • Paper • ISBN 0-89594-781-1

## Healing with Chinese Herbs

By Lesley Tierra

Tierra lists the properties and therapeutic uses of over one hundred herbs. Includes a glossary of Chinese terms, an index to the Latin and Mandarin names of each herb, and guidelines to dosages.

$14.95 • Paper • ISBN 0-89594-829-X

## Healthy Parents, Better Babies

By Francesca Naish and Janette Roberts

Did you know that the food you eat, the environment you line in, and the lifestyle you lead in the months before you conceive a child can have a profound effect on the well-being of your baby? The book is a complete, easy to follow guide to optimal preconception health for both prospective parents.

$16.95 • Paper • ISBN 0-89594-955-5

## The Herbal Menopause Book: *Herbs, Nutrition, and Other Natural Therapies*

By Amanda McQuade Crawford

This comprehensive volume provides dozens of specific herbal remedies and other natural therapies for women facing the health issues that arise in premenopause, menopause, and post menopause.

$16.95 • Paper • ISBN 0-89594-799-4

# RELATED BOOKS BY THE CROSSING PRESS

## The Herbs of Life: *Health & Healing Using Western & Chinese Techniques*

By Lesley Tierra

"This book is an herbalist's delight! It combines Western, Chinese, and Ayurvedic tradition with emphasis on energy patterns of illness and corresponding energies of herbs and food." —The American Herb Association

$16.95 • Paper • ISBN 0-89594-498-7

## The Information Sourcebook of Herbal Medicine

By David Hoffman, B.Sc., M.N.I.M.H.

A comprehensive guide to information on western herbal medicine, offering a bibliography of herbalism and herbal pharmacology, a glossary of herbal and medical terms, computer databases for the herbalist, and Medline citations for commonly used medicinal herbs.

$40.00 • Hardcover • ISBN 0-89594-671-8

## The Male Herbal: *Health Care for Men & Boys*

By James Green

This preventive health care guide offers remedies for specific male problems, information on choosing the right herb, and preparation of herbal medicines.

$14.95 • Paper • ISBN 0-89594-458-8

## Natural Healing for Babies & Children

By Aviva Jill Romm

This is an indispensable volume for parents seeking safe and effective ways to promote and maintain their child's health using herbal and other natural remedies.

$16.95 • Paper • ISBN 0-89594-786-2

## The Natural Remedy Book for Women

By Diane Stein

This bestselling, self-help guide to holistic health care includes information on ten different natural healing methods. Remedies from all ten methods are given for fifty common health problems.

$16.95 • Paper • ISBN 0-89594-525-8

# RELATED BOOKS BY THE CROSSING PRESS

## The Optimum Nutrition Bible
By Patrick Holford

Optimum nutrition is a revolution in health care. It means giving yourself the best possible intake of nutrients to allow your body to be as healthy as possible. This book shows you precisely how to achieve this.

$16.95 • Paper • ISBN 1-58091-015-7

## Pocket Guide to Aromatherapy
By Kathi Keville

In use for more than 600 years, aromatherapy offers a powerful tool for physical and emotional healing. This guide includes a list of the best essential oils for each particular condition, tips on making your own formulas, and special sections on first-aid, childhood problems and emotional well-being.

$6.95 • Paper • ISBN 0-89594-815-X

## Pocket Guide to Ayurvedic Healing
By Candis Cantin Packard

Widely practiced in India, Ayurveda (the "science of life") combines physical, psychological, and spiritual therapies in a holistic approach to health. This is a concise guide to this ancient healing art and includes an overview of Ayurvedic principles, self-diagnostic tests, simple herbal remedies and ayurvedic case studies.

$6.95 • Paper • ISBN 0-89594-764-1

## Pocket Guide to Bach Flower Essences
By Rachelle Hasnas

Bach flower essences provide a remarkable form of energetic healing for yourself, your family and pets. You can learn how to select appropriate flower essences with confidence and use them to bring your body, mind and spirit into harmony.

$6.95 • Paper • ISBN 0-89594-865-6

## Pocket Guide to Chinese Patent Medicines
By Bill Schoenbart, L.Ac.

This handy guide organizes Chinese Patent Medicines according to organ systems and diagnostic categories. Each medicine description includes the illnesses associated with its cure, ingredients, dosage, manufacturer, and any contraindications that may apply.

$6.95 • Paper • ISBN 0-89594-978-4

# Related Books by The Crossing Press

## Pocket Guide to Macrobiotics
By Carl Ferré

Benefits of a Macrobiotics regime include less fatigue, relief from pain and illness, renewed enjoyment of food, more fulfilling sex life, better sleep, and improved memory and clearer thinking.

$6.95 • Paper • ISBN 0-89594-848-6

## Pocket Guide to Naturopathic Medicine
By Judith Boice

Combining the best current medical practice with remedies of the past, naturopathic medicine works to enhance your body's innate healing capacity. This guide includes therapy for allergies, skin conditions, digestive problems, menstrual cramping and children's illnesses.

$6.95 • Paper • ISBN 0-89594-821-4

## Pocket Guide to Stress Reduction
By Brenda O'Hanlon

This take-along guide provides a useful checklist to assess your stress level and teaches you various ways to reduce your stress. Learn how to manage, harness and control the stress in your life rather than allowing it to control you.

$6.95 • Paper • ISBN 0-58091-011-4

## Pocket Herbal Reference Guide
By Debra St. Claire

The medicinal use of plants is our oldest form of healing. This guide describes the appropriate use of herbs in an easily referenced format, including the therapeutic use of over 140 medicinal plants and natural remedies for over 100 common health problems.

$6.95 • Paper • ISBN 0-89594-568-1

## Rejuvenate: *A 21-Day Natural Detox Plan for Optimal Health*
By Helene Silver

Rejuvenate will show you how you can create a retreat for yourself in the comfort and privacy of your own home. With step-by-step instructions, Silver's 21-day plan will cleanse your body of toxins and rejuvenate both body and mind.

$16.95 • Paper • ISBN 0-89594-938-5